An Atlas of
HAIR AND
SCALP DISEASES

THE ENCYCLOPEDIA OF VISUAL MEDICINE SERIES

An Atlas of
HAIR AND
SCALP DISEASES

J. Powell, N. Stone and R.P.R. Dawber

Dermatology Department
The Oxford Radcliffe Hospital
Headington, Oxford, UK

The Parthenon Publishing Group
International Publishers in Medicine, Science & Technology

A CRC PRESS COMPANY
BOCA RATON   LONDON   NEW YORK   WASHINGTON, D.C.

Published in the USA by
The Parthenon Publishing Group Inc.
One Blue Hill Plaza
PO Box 1564
Pearl River
New York 10965
USA

Published in the UK by
The Parthenon Publishing Group
23–25 Blades Court
Deodar Road
London SW15 2NU
UK

Copyright © 2002 The Parthenon Publishing Group

Library of Congress Cataloging-in-Publication Data

Powell, J. (Jennifer), 1955-
    An atlas of hair and scalp diseases / J. Powell, N. Stone, and R.P.R. Dawber.
        p. ; cm. -- (Encyclopedia of visual medicine series)
    Includes bibliographical references and index.
    ISBN 1-84214-013-2 (alk. paper)
        1. Hair--Diseases--Atlases. 2. Scalp--Diseases--Atlases. I. Stone, N. (Natalie), 1967-
II. Dawber, R.P.R. (Rodney P.R.) III. Title. IV. Series.
        [DNLM: 1. Hair Diseases--Atlases. 2. Head and Neck Neoplasms--Atlases. 3.
Scalp--Atlases. 4. Scalp Dermatoses--Atlases. 5. Skin Neoplasms--Atlases. WR 17
P884a 2001]
    RL151.P69 2001
    616.5′46′00222--dc21   2001036103

British Library Cataloguing in Publication Data

Powell, J.
    An atlas of hair and scalp diseases. - (The encyclopedia of visual medicine series)
    1. Hair - Diseases 2. Scalp - Diseases
    I. Title II. Stone, N. III. Dawber R.P.R. (Rodney P.R.)
    616.5′46

ISBN 1-84214-013-2

First published in 2002

Composition by The Parthenon Publishing Group
Color reproduction by Graphic Reproductions, UK
Printed and bound by T. G. Hostench S.A., Spain

Contents

Preface

Abnormalities of the hair are immediately apparent and all doctors are faced with patients suffering with these problems. Dermatologists and primary-care physicians see many patients specifically seeking help with such disorders. In this situation, it is useful to have access to a comprehensive but simple collection of physical signs with concise guidance as to their significance.

Hair is not essential for health and survival in humans as it is in other mammals. Despite this, changes in its growth density, pattern or alterations in its color and texture often lead to great distress in the patient. In addition, they may indicate underlying systemic disease including endocrine, genetic, metabolic or nutritional and psychiatric disorders.

This Atlas attempts to illustrate the enormous range of changes in hair and its growth. Over 200 carefully selected illustrations are accompanied by concise clinical information on diagnosis, practical management, and recent advances in our knowledge and understanding of each disorder.

In nine chapters, we have illustrated the basic physiology of hair growth, congenital and hair shaft abnormalities, including cosmetic damage to hair, loss and overgrowth of hair, and abnormalities of the scalp, including inflammatory, infective and malignant skin disease.

This new Atlas will provide an important resource for education, reference and management for all physicians. Hair and scalp diseases may not be life-threatening but they are widespread and cause much distress to many patients. We hope that, by increasing the ability of readers to recognize and diagnose these conditions and improving the management of them, this book will help both physician and patient.

1

Characteristics of hair development, structure and growth

INTRODUCTION

Hair is a characteristic of mammals. Many species that have a general covering of hair depend on it for conserving heat and camouflage. Molting allows for seasonal variation of weight and color of the coat. In humans, hair is not essential for survival but is important in individual recognition and in sexual attraction. Also, although Man has lost the general covering of hair, the number of hair follicles per unit area of skin remains as high or higher than in other mammals. Hair forms part of our mechanism of light–touch sensation.

HAIR DEVELOPMENT AND EMBRYOLOGY

An examination of hair embryology helps to understand the cycle of growth of hair and the hair shaft structure. Development of hair follicles starts at 9–12 weeks of gestation. On the upper lip, chin and eyebrow regions (areas of specialized sensory 'vibrissa' hairs in many lower animals), widespread follicle development begins in the 4th month. First, a crowding of cells occurs in the fetal basal layer cells of the epidermis (as a result of a signal from the underlying dermis – shown in recombinant studies where chick dermis can instruct mouse epidermis to produce a feather rather than a hair and vice versa). These cells elongate and grow downwards as a 'hair peg' (Figure 1.1a). The concave end carries a group of mesenchymal cells that become the dermal papilla and the root sheath (Figure 1.1b). The dermal papilla cells become enclosed by the hair peg and form the matrix from which the hair and inner root sheath develop (Figures 1.1c and d). This population of cells

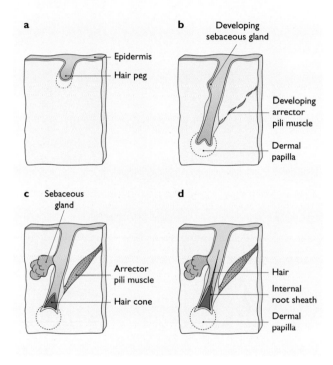

Figure 1.1

remains stable throughout successive adult hair cycles.

HAIR STRUCTURE

Rapidly dividing cells in the hair matrix differentiate into a variety of cell types. They arrange into concentric layers and undergo phases of hardening and keratinization (with cell death). The three innermost layers form the definitive hair shaft: medulla, cortex and cuticle. These layers can be seen in diagrams

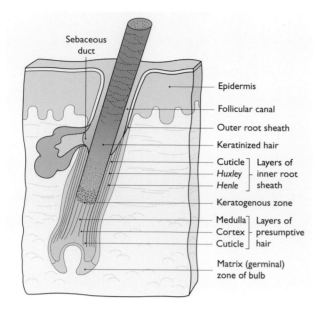

Figure 1.2

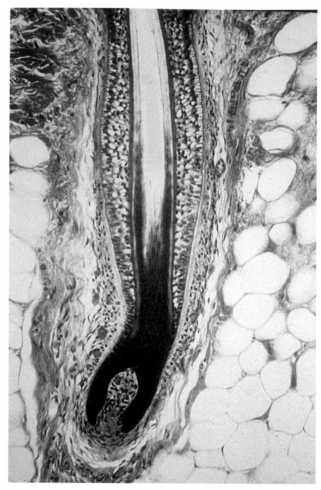

Figure 1.4

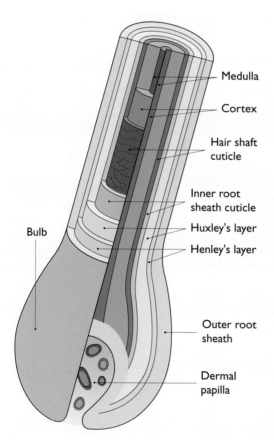

Figure 1.3

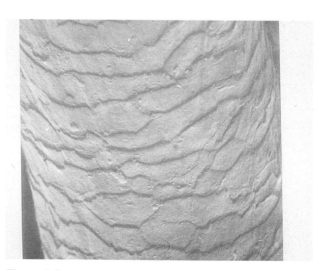

Figure 1.5

both longitudinal (Figure 1.2) and transverse (Figure 1.3) and also in histological sections of the scalp (Figure 1.4).

The medullary cells are large and spherical, and are found in the core of some terminal hairs with air spaces between and within them. Cortical cells form the bulk of the hair shaft and become closely packed, interdigitating longitudinally with orientated spindle-shaped cells. These produce cytoplasmic filaments parallel to the long axis of the cell and hair

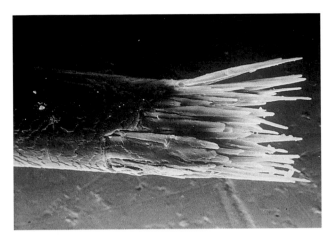

Figure 1.6

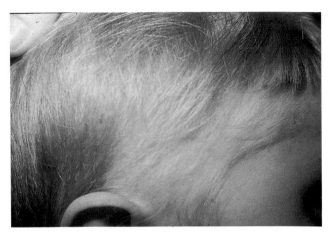

Figure 1.7

shaft. Surface cuticular cells, rich in high-density sulfur protein, elongate and flatten, and overlap from root to tip like roof tiles (Figure 1.5). This hair structure is very stable, having evolved to withstand external physical forces. It stays intact even thousands of years after death, although evidence of natural 'weathering' may be found microscopically, especially in the distal ends of longer hairs (Figure 1.6).

The inner root sheath hardens before the hair within it. This protects the developing hair and defines its shape, bore and diameter. The 'bore' or cross-section of the hair varies with race and with disease. Mongoloid hair is circular and very straight, Negroid hair is oval and curled and subject to increased weathering, while Caucasoid hair is variable, but typically ovoid and wavy. The outer root sheath is a sleeve of differentiated epidermis continuous with that on the scalp. A connective tissue sheath surrounds the structure, also enclosing the sebaceous gland and duct, the arrector pili muscle (which attaches at the 'bulge' of the follicle, the possible stem cell zone), and the rich vascular and nervous supplies.

HAIR TYPES

Initially, 'lanugo' hair is formed. This is fine and non-medullated and typically shed *in utero* in the 8th month of gestation (see Chapter 2, Figure 2.7). The second shorter lanugo growth is shed at 3–4 months postnatally, usually imperceptibly as a molt because the hair growth is synchronized. Postnatal hair is divided into two groups, vellus and terminal, and is shed in unsynchronized fashion. Vellus hair is short, fine, non-medullated and lightly pigmented (Figure 1.7). Some types of terminal hair are thick, long, medullated and pigmented. In children, terminal hairs occur only on the scalp, eyebrows and lashes, but at puberty many vellus hairs become terminal under the influence of androgens. Meanwhile, paradoxically, some terminal hairs on the scalp may miniaturize and become vellus-like hairs beyond puberty (androgenetic alopecia or common baldness). Some types of terminal hair are shown in Figures 1.12–1.15.

THE HAIR CYCLE

The hair follicle does not grow continuously like the epidermis, but undergoes a repetitive cycle of growth (the anagen phase), involution (the catagen phase) and rest (the telogen phase). This can be seen histologically in Figure 1.8 (anagen) and Figure 1.9 (catagen) and also in plucked hairs. (Figure 1.10a shows the anagen phase and Figure 1.10b the telogen phase.) Linear hair growth rate is approximately 1 cm per month on the scalp. The length of hair attained is governed largely by the length of phases of the hair cycle. Anagen lasts 3–5 years, catagen approximately 5 weeks, and telogen 3–5 months. On the normal scalp, 80–90% of the 100 000 hair follicles on the scalp are in the anagen phase, and 12–15% in the telogen phase. This means that 100–150 hairs are normally lost per day. The hair cycle (Figure 1.11) is not synchronized, so molting does not occur and, in healthy subjects, the density of scalp hair remains largely unchanged.

Anagen development of a new hair follicle repeats the morphogenesis described in fetal skin. As catagen approaches, mitosis in the matrix ceases and

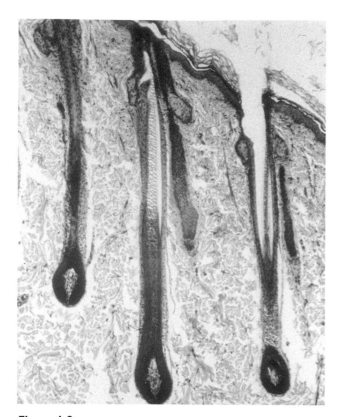

Figure 1.8

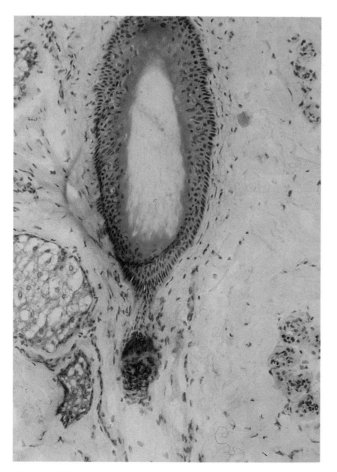

Figure 1.9

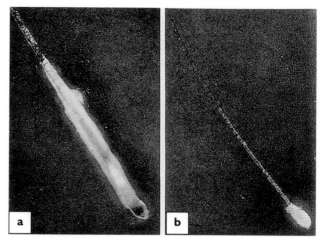

Figure 1.10

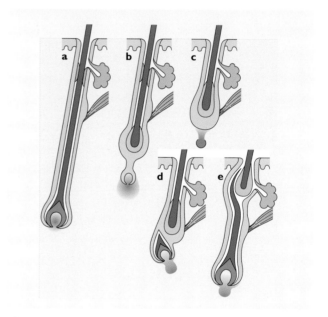

Figure 1.11

the hair root becomes club-shaped. It also becomes colorless because melanization ceases. The outer root sheath undergoes apoptotic degeneration, and the club hair moves upwards to lie at the level of insertion of the arrector muscle. During telogen, the resting phase, the club is held in an epithelial sac, with the dermal papilla as a ball of 'inactive' cells underlying it. The follicle re-enters anagen spontaneously (the mechanism for re-activation remains uncertain) or may be induced to do so if the resting hair is plucked.

Each hair follicle is controlled by the dermal papilla, but overall control of the hair cycle is complex. In childhood, a greater proportion of hair follicles are in the anagen phase, and at puberty this changes to, and stabilizes at, approximately 12% of

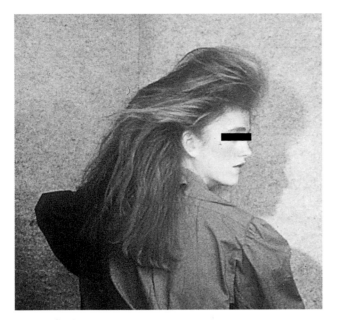

Figure 1.12

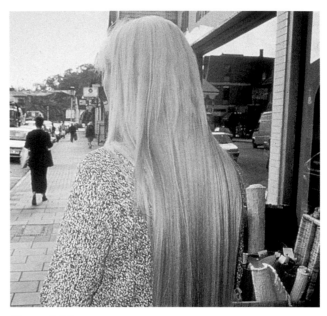

Figure 1.14

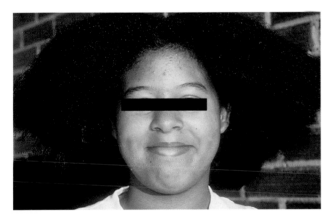

Figure 1.13
Reproduced with kind permission of Dr John Gray and first published in
Human Hair Diversity, by Blackwells, Oxford, 2000

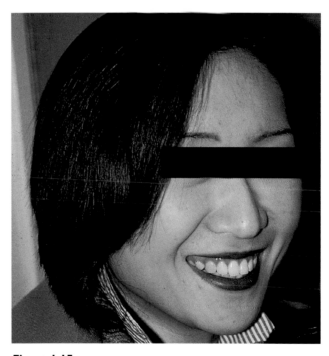

Figure 1.15
Reproduced with kind permission of Dr John Gray and first published in
Human Hair Diversity, by Blackwells, Oxford, 2000

hairs being in the telogen phase. With age or illness, the anagen phase shortens, leading to increased daily shedding and shorter maximum length of the hairs. Hair growth is affected by local growth factors and hormonal influences, especially androgens, in addition to complex genetic, racial and sexual factors. Racial differences may be seen in Figures 1.12–1.15: red hair in a Celtic-skinned female (Figure 1.12), AfroCaribbean hair (Figure 1.13), long fair hair in a Caucasian (Figure 1.14), and Asian hair (Figure 1.15). These racial differences may also be seen in cross-sections of the hairs. Light micrographs of hairs show Asian hair to be circular in cross-section, while Caucasian hairs are oval and AfroCaribbean hairs are almost flattened (Figure 1.16). Differences

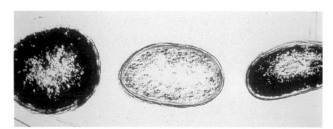

Figure 1.16

between individuals may also be explained by variations in receptivity and reactivity of the hair follicles to external and hormonal factors.

REFERENCES

1. Dawber RPR. *Diseases of the Hair and Scalp*, 3rd edn. Oxford: Blackwell Science, 1997:1–50

2. Hardy MH. The secret life of the hair follicle. *Trends Genet* 1992;8:55

3. Hashimoto K. Structure of human hair. *Clin Dermatol* 1988;6:4

4. Gillespie JM. The structural proteins of hair: isolation, characterization and regulation of biosynthesis. In Goldsmith LA, ed. *Biochemistry and Physiology of Skin*, Volume 1. Oxford: Oxford University Press, 1983:475

2

Congenital disorders of the hair and scalp

ALOPECIA

Occipital alopecia of the newborn

In the first 2 months of life, infants commonly develop a temporary patch of alopecia over the occiput. Hair grows in two waves following birth (Figure 2.1), with hair from the first wave predominating at the occiput. In this region, hair does not initially enter the telogen phase of the cycle and is lost in a synchronized manner leading to this area of alopecia, a loss that is exacerbated by friction from rubbing. Hair growth is normal in this site by 1 year of age.

Atrichia congenita

This is a rare condition where the absence of scalp hair is total and permanent (Figure 2.2). Several distinct genodermatoses share this feature.

Inheritance is usually autosomal recessive, but autosomal dominant types also occur. Scalp hair is usually absent at birth and, if it is initially present, it is shed in the first 6 months and fails to regrow. Hair growth can be normal for up to 5 years before permanent loss occurs. Histologically, hair follicles are almost completely absent but a few small, thin hairs of normal structure can remain. Atrichia congenita is often an isolated finding, but may be associated with other ectodermal defects or form part of a separate syndrome.

Hypotrichosis

Hypotrichosis is the partial absence of scalp hair (Figure 2.3). It may be an isolated finding, the so-

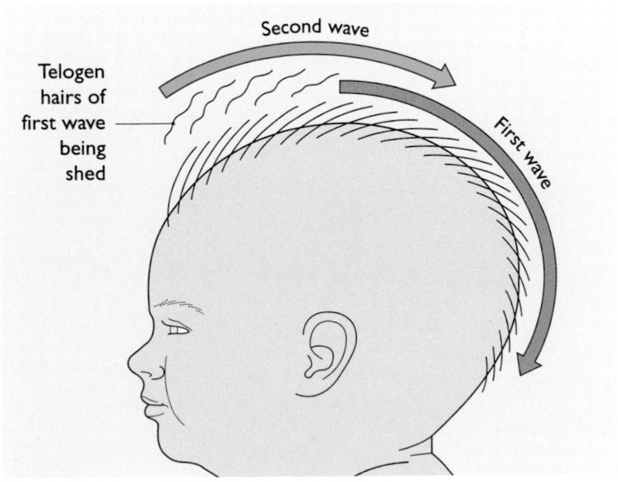

Figure 2.1

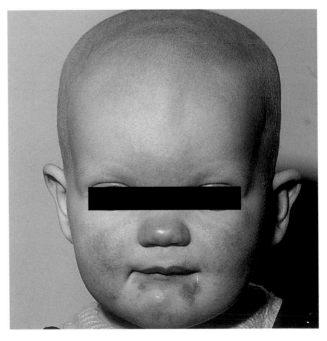

Figure 2.2

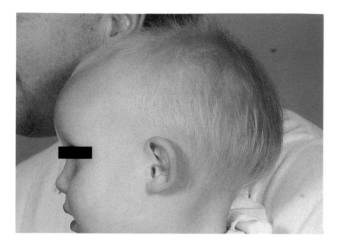

Figure 2.3

called hypotrichosis simplex. It can also be associated with other ectodermal defects, of which there are numerous examples, or it may be part of a separate syndrome or disease, including the basal cell carcinoma syndromes, Basex and Rombo, chromosomal syndromes such as Down's, Klinefelter's and Turner's, the premature aging syndromes of progeria and Werner's, xeroderma pigmentosum, Cockayne's syndrome, Rothmund–Thomson syndrome, and acrodermatitis enteropathica.

The hair shafts can either be normal in structure or display a distinctive defect such as is seen in pili torti or Netherton's syndrome (see Chapter 5). Hair growth can be normal at birth but hair is often shed at 6 months and regrowth is poor. It is important to examine the patient and his/her relatives for other ectodermal defects.

Marie–Unna hypotrichosis

This is a distinct, autosomal dominant form of hypotrichosis in which patients may be born with sparse or normal hair which is lost in infancy; hair growth recurs around 3 years of age. Hair shafts of this new growth are characteristically coarse and twisted and have a similar wiry feel to horse hair (Figure 2.4a), giving the overall appearance of a cheap wig. Patchy, progressive hair loss then occurs from puberty onwards (Figure 2.4b). There are usually no other associated features and there is no treatment.

Aplasia cutis congenita

Aplasia cutis congenita of the scalp presents as scarred, depressed areas of alopecia, due to aplasia of

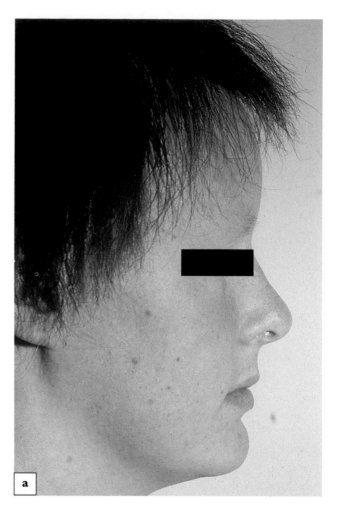

a

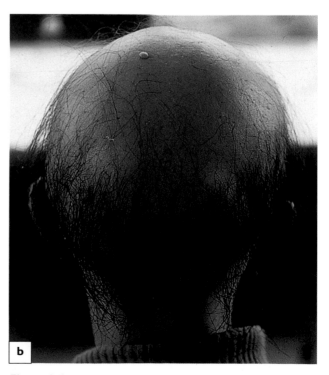

b

Figure 2.4

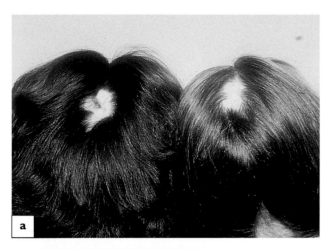

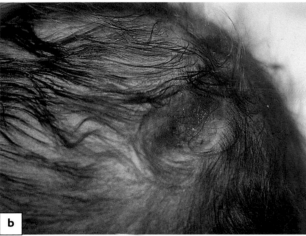

Figure 2.5

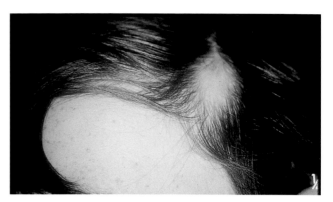

Figure 2.6

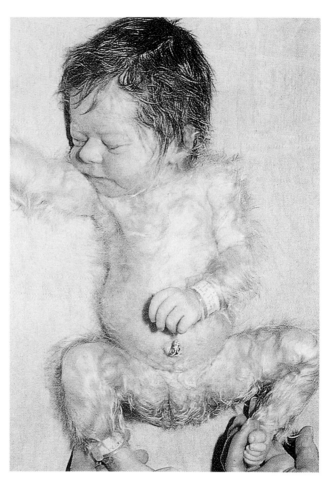

Figure 2.7

all skin layers (Figure 2.5a). It has been reported in association with many different abnormalities, including anomalous veins, limb abnormalities and epidermal nevi. It is clinically important that neuroectodermal defects, such as encephaloceles or heterotropic brain tissue, may present with a similar clinical appearance. Such neuroectodermal defects may be more likely to be surrounded by a collar of hypertrophic hair – the 'hair collar' sign (Figure 2.5b) and they may overlie cranial defects. All these lesions should therefore be investigated radiologically prior to intervention.

Triangular alopecia

Triangular alopecia is a non-scarring, triangle-shaped area of alopecia, usually unilateral and overlying the frontotemporal suture (Figure 2.6). The area is permanent but non-progressive. Parents usually only notice the area of alopecia when the child is aged 3–6 years. It is relatively common and no treatment is required.

HYPERTRICHOSIS

Congenital hypertrichosis lanuginosa

Hypertrichosis lanuginosa is an extremely rare condition in which the whole body, excluding palms and soles, is covered by long, silky, lanugo hair (Figure 2.7). The abnormality is usually present at birth but can develop later. Hair growth may become less dense with time but is usually retained.

Congenital hypertrichosis

Severe forms of congenital hypertrichosis have been reported. Patients are born with coarse terminal hair, particularly in the facial area (Figure 2.8). An X-linked dominant inheritance has been described.

Focal lumbosacral hypertrichosis

Focal lumbosacral hypertrichosis is also known as faun tail or 'false tail', a nevoid area of lanugo hair in the lumbosacral region (Figure 2.9). It is present at birth and is retained. It is often a sign of an underlying spinal dysraphism. Full neurologic and radiologic investigation of these cases is important.

PIGMENTATION

Poliosis

Poliosis is a localized patch of white hair due to a deficiency in melanogenesis (Figure 2.10). The defect is the same in the follicle and the surrounding epidermis. A white forelock can have an autosomal dominant inheritance as part of the disorder called piebaldism, which results from a defect in the kit proto-oncogene. Poliosis may also be associated with tuberous sclerosis, where it may be the presenting sign.

Albinism

In oculocutaneous albinism, melanocytes are present in normal numbers but melanin production is impaired, so the skin, eyes and hair appear 'colorless'. Hair is usually yellow but can appear to have a reddish tinge (Figure 2.11).

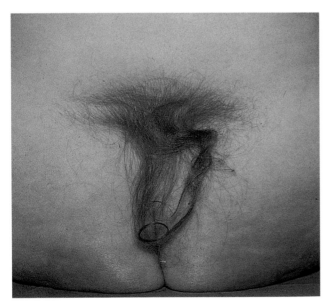

Figure 2.8

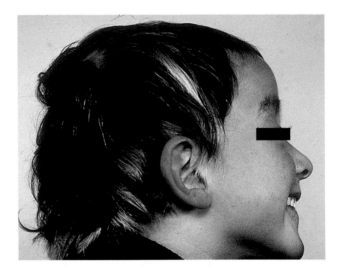

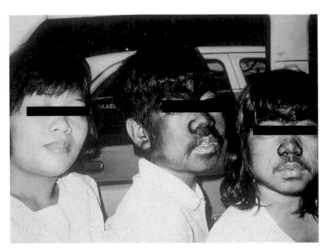

Figure 2.9

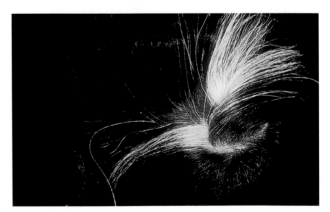

Figure 2.10

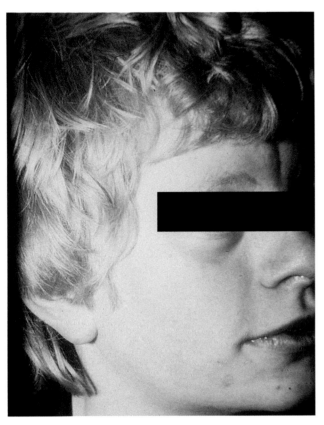

Figure 2.11

REFERENCES

1. Bently-Philips B, Grace HJ. Hereditary hypotrichosis. *Br J Dermatol* 1979;101:331

2. Unna M. Uber Hypotrichosis congenita hereditaria. *Dermatol Wochenschrift* 1925;81:1167

3. Commens C, Rogers M, Kan A. Heterotropic brain tissue presenting as a bald cyst with a collar of hypertropic hair. *Arch Dermatol* 1989;125:1253

4. Drolet B, Prendiville J, Golden J, *et al*. Membranous aplasia cutis with hair collars. *Arch Dermatol* 1995;131:1427–31

5. Tosti A. Congenital triangular alopecia. *J Am Acad Dermatol* 1987;16:991

6. Sinclair R, de Berker D. Hereditary and congenital hypotrichosis. In Dawber RPR, ed. *Diseases of the Hair and Scalp*. Oxford: Blackwell Science, 1997:151–238

7. Partridge JW. Congenital hypertrichosis lanuginosa: neonatal shaving. *Arch Dis Childhood* 1987;62:623

8. Macias-Flores MA, Garcia-Cruz D, Rivera H, *et al*. A new form of hypertrichosis inherited as an X-linked dominant trait. *Hum Genetics* 1984;66:66

9. Tomita Y. The molecular basis of albinism and piebaldism. *Arch Dermatol* 1994;130:355

3

Alopecia

ALOPECIA AREATA

Alopecia areata is a condition of unknown etiology causing isolated patches of baldness on the scalp of healthy individuals, adults (Figure 3.1) or children (Figure 3.2). This pattern gives a good prognosis for regrowth (if limited to one to three patches, spontaneous regrowth in 1 year is likely). It is quite common, with 1% of the population affected with it by the age of 55 years. For alopecia areata occurring in childhood or adolescence, the incidence peaks at age 4–5 years. Thirty-five percent of those patients in whom the onset of the disease occurs before age 20 years have a family history of alopecia areata. There is an increased incidence of atopy in patients and family members, and also of autoimmune disease (thyroiditis, vitiligo, diabetes mellitus, pernicious anemia, Addison's disease) and of associated auto-antibodies in patients and family members.

The area of bald scalp in alopecia areata may appear peach-colored, and there may be a positive 'pull test' if the condition is active (hairs come out abnormally easily if pulled gently). At the margins of

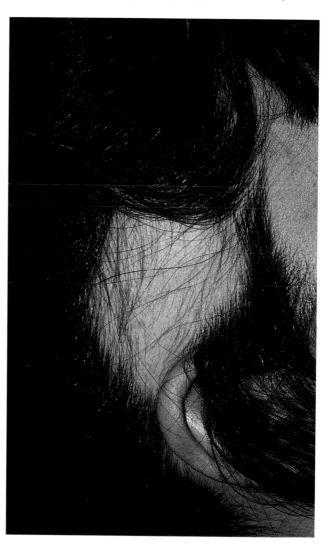

Figure 3.2

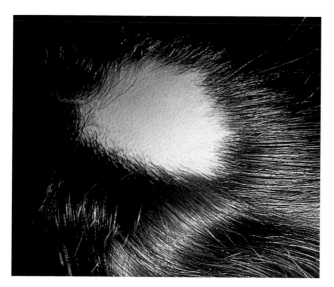

Figure 3.1

active lesions, there may be pathognomonic 'exclamation mark' hairs (Figure 3.3), which signify the area of 'activity'. These are of normal width at the tip but narrow at the base, a phenomenon that becomes more obvious when the hair is plucked (Figure 3.4). The telogen root has a narrow section of non-pigmented hair immediately above, but distally it becomes wider and darker.

Areas other than the scalp may be affected by alopecia areata. Eyebrows (Figure 3.5) and eyelashes (Figure 3.6) are quite frequently totally or partially lost. It may also affect sites on the trunk and limbs, the central chest (Figure 3.7), or the beard area, where the resulting pallor may be misdiagnosed as hypopigmentation (Figure 3.8).

A reticulate patchy type of alopecia areata (Figure 3.9) may precede the onset of the loss of all hair on the scalp (alopecia totalis), or all hair on the body (alopecia universalis). Rapid progression to diffuse shedding (Figure 3.10) may also signify progression to alopecia totalis (Figure 3.11). A number of other factors predict a poor prognosis for the regrowth of hair (and make persistent alopecia totalis more likely). These are the onset of alopecia totalis before puberty, a pattern of loss at the scalp margins (ophiasis) (Figure 3.12), multiple lesions (especially those away from the scalp) and associated

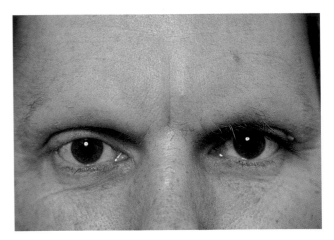

Figure 3.5

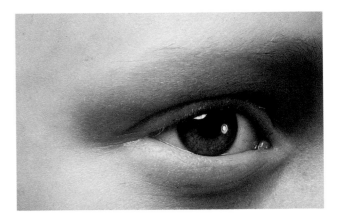

Figure 3.6

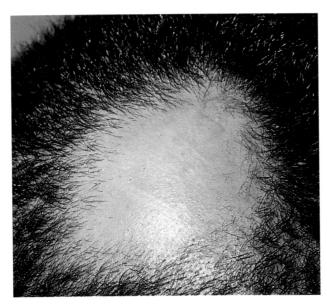

Figure 3.3

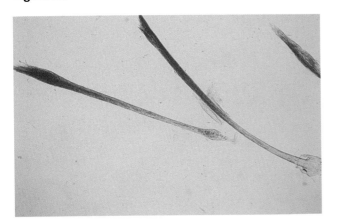

Figure 3.4

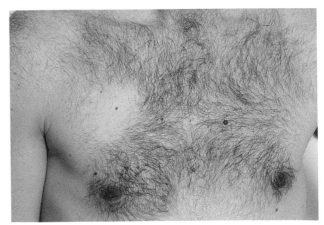

Figure 3.7

Down's syndrome (Figure 3.13). There is also a positive association with atopy, but this does not appear to affect the prognosis.

The hair loss in alopecia areata preferentially affects pigmented hairs, and regrowth is often unpigmented in both young (Figure 3.14) and older age groups (Figure 3.15). Rapid onset of alopecia areata may give the appearance of 'going white overnight

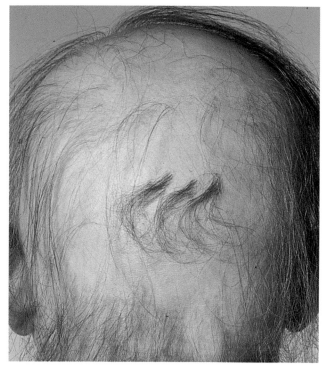

Figure 3.10

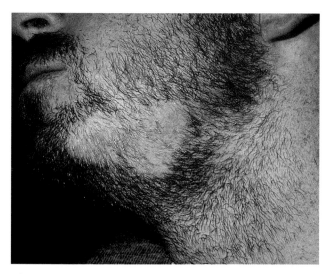

Figure 3.8

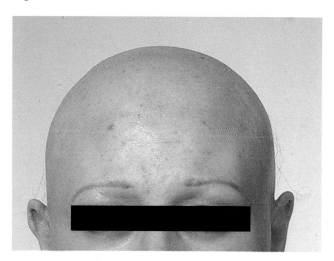

Figure 3.11

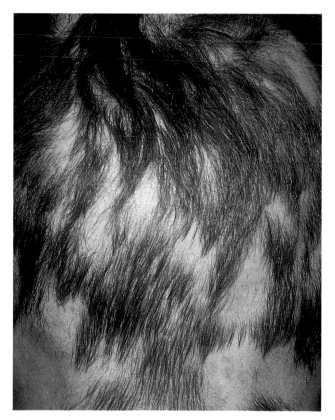

Figure 3.9

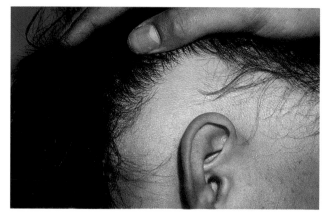

Figure 3.12

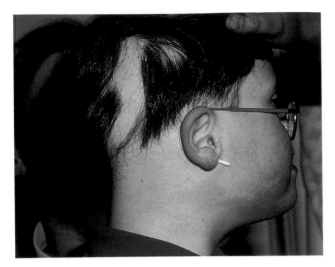

Figure 3.13

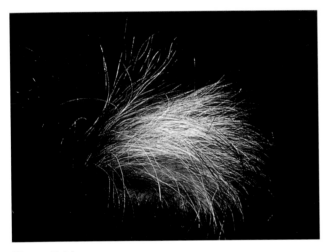

Figure 3.14

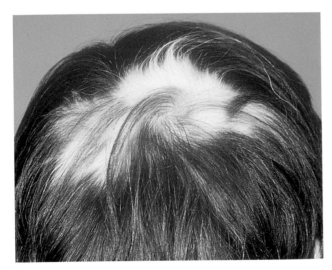

Figure 3.15

owing to shock' as colored hairs are lost, leaving only white ones. Stress is often linked to the onset of the hair loss, but its role in etiology remains uncertain. Similarly, in alopecia totalis, all the scalp hairs are lost, but, if the scalp is viewed against a dark background, regrowth of fine depigmented hairs is seen (Figure 3.16). Histological examination of a hair follicle in an area of scalp with alopecia areata shows a 'swarm' of lymphocytes around affected anagen follicles (Figure 3.17). Nail deformities may be seen in association with, or they may precede the hair loss in, alopecia areata. Thinning, pitting and dystrophy of the nail may be seen (Figure 3.18). Despite many theories as to its etiology, management of alopecia areata remains difficult. It is important to explain the disorder and inform the patient of the natural course of the disease. The majority of patients (exact percentages vary with different reports) improve spontaneously. Others carry a poor prognosis for regrowth. Many patients will choose to have no treatment. If there is less than 50% loss, topical and intralesional steroids may be useful. Topical minoxi-

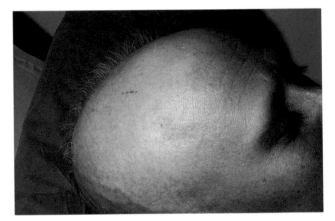

Figure 3.16

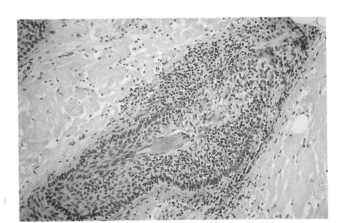

Figure 3.17

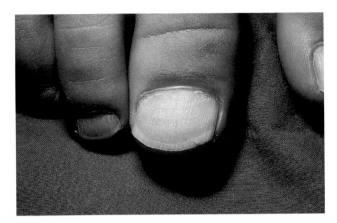

Figure 3.18

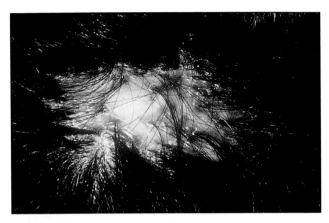

Figure 3.19

dil may help if there is some residual hair. Short contact irritant or allergen therapy may give some regrowth, but this is temporary and risks sensitizing not only the patient but the nurses and carers also. If there is over 50% loss, some patients will require a wig or tattoos of the eyebrows. Other options are systemic steroids, cyclosporin or psoralen and ultra-violet A therapy.

CICATRICIAL ALOPECIA (SCARRING ALOPECIA)

Cicatricial alopecia occurs when there is destruction of the hair follicles. There may be an obvious cause such as a developmental fault, trauma such as burns, encroachment of a tumor, infection or a scarring dermatosis. In some cases, the cause may not become apparent. It is important to examine the skin of the scalp and elsewhere for other signs, and systemic investigations may be necessary. Scarring is not always easy to identify clinically, and it may be necessary to re-examine the patient after an interval, or to take a biopsy from the margin of a recently affected area, although histology does not always provide a diagnostic answer.

Folliculitis decalvans and tufted folliculitis

Folliculitis decalvans is a crusted and pustular infection of the scalp that leads to patches of permanent alopecia with follicular scarring (Figure 3.19). The bacterium *Staphylococcus aureus* is found on culture. Short courses of antibiotics are not helpful, and, during long courses, the condition may relapse. Certain combinations of antibiotics over several months have been shown to be helpful in some

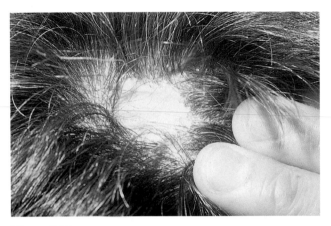

Figure 3.20

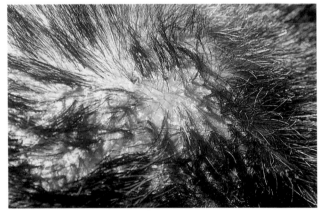

Figure 3.21

patients (rifampicin and clindamycin together orally). After treatment, although the scarred alopecia persists, the area is free from pustules and inflammation, and symptoms of soreness improve (Figure 3.20).

In tufted folliculitis, on a background of pustular inflammation and scarring alopecia, 'tufts' of hairs may be seen emerging together through one follicular opening (Figure 3.21). The presentation, course and prognosis do not differ from those of folliculitis decalvans. Tufting may be seen in other forms of scarring of the scalp, and may reflect a more superficial level of inflammation and scarring, destroying the exit route for the hair while leaving the deeper part of the follicle unharmed.

Lichen planus

Patients with lichen planus of the scalp have patches of dull red follicular inflammation which produce enlarging areas of scarring alopecia (Figure 3.22). Occasionally, the pattern of lichen plano-pilaris is seen (Figure 3.23). This form of lichen planus is centered around the hair follicles and it may cause rapid-onset and permanent alopecia. There may be lesions of lichen planus on the skin elsewhere to aid in making a diagnosis. These include typical violaceous, polygonal, pruritic papules with superficial white streaks (Wickham's striae) often seen on the wrists (Figure 3.24), and typical white lacy lesions on the buccal mucosa (Figure 3.25). There may also be painful erosive lesions and the nails may be dystrophic and thinned (Figure 3.26). A biopsy may be necessary to give diagnostic histology (Figure 3.27). This histologic section is stained with H & E

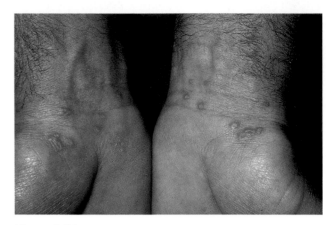

Figure 3.24

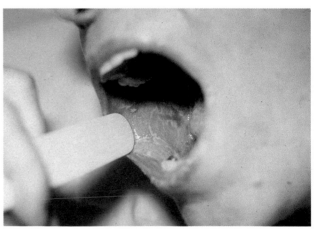

Figure 3.25

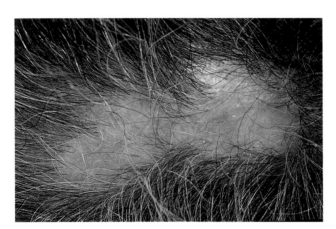

Figure 3.22

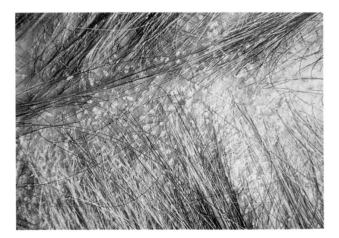

Figure 3.23

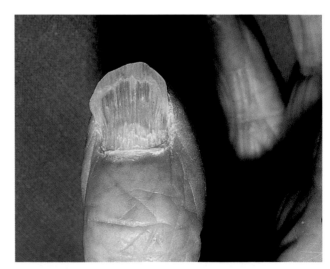

Figure 3.26

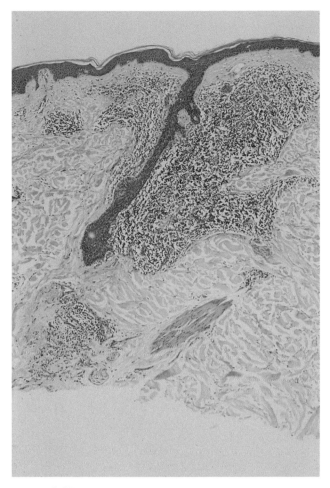

Figure 3.27

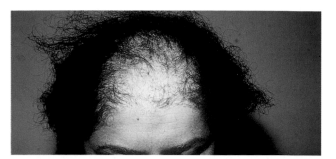

Figure 3.28

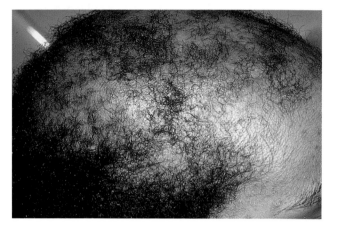

Figure 3.29

to show a subepidermal band-like inflammatory infiltrate and some basal cell degenerative changes, with cytoid bodies. It is important to exclude any drugs or chemicals that may be causing the lichenoid reaction in the skin, and treatment is usually with potent topical or intralesional corticosteroids to reduce any active inflammation. In more severe cases, oral steroids or other immunosuppressive drugs such as azathioprine and cyclosporin may be considered.

Frontal fibrosing alopecia

Patients with lichen planus-type cicatricial alopecia affecting mainly the frontal area of the scalp make up a distinct clinical group (Figure 3.28). They do not have the associated skin, mucosal and nail changes of lichen planus. In black African patients, a similar entity named follicular degeneration syndrome is recognized (Figure 3.29).

Lupus erythematosus

Lupus erythematosus is an autoimmune disorder which may be systemic (SLE), affecting the skin and the internal organs, or 'discoid' (DLE) affecting the skin alone. Scalp changes are frequent in both types. Alopecia occurs in 50% of cases of acute SLE (often associated with facial erythema in the form of a 'butterfly' rash). There may be some erythema of the scalp, and diffuse shedding of the hair; any hairs left may be fragile and short.

DLE usually begins on the face, but scalp lesions develop in 20% of male and 50% of female patients. Erythema and scaling extend irregularly to leave obvious scarring of both the face and the scalp with alopecia (Figure 3.30). It may also be transferred across the placenta to cause transient neonatal lupus erythematosus (Figure 3.31). DLE occurring in dark-skinned patients (Figure 3.32) may cause scarring alopecia with loss of pigment, and surrounding hyperpigmented inflammation with follicular plugging (hyperkeratosis at the site of each hair follicle).

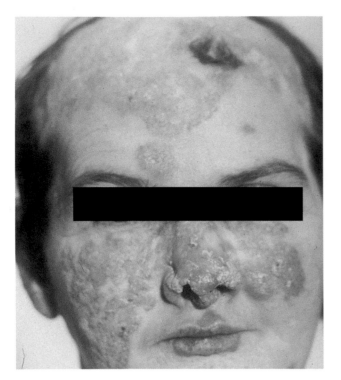

Figure 3.30

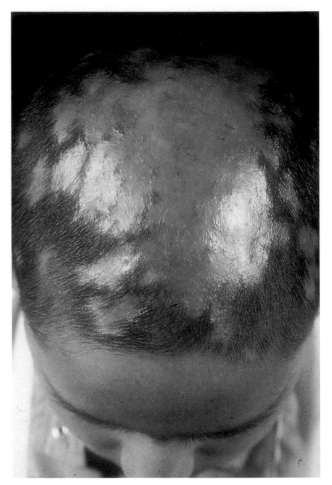

Figure 3.32

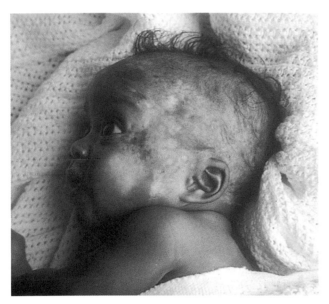

Figure 3.31

Pseudopelade

Pseudopelade, translated literally, means mimicking alopecia areata, but is caused by a progressive loss of follicles with scarring alopecia, without any clinically obvious inflammation. The cause is unknown, but it may represent a specific autoimmune disease, or a non-specific end-stage of lichen planus or lupus erythematosus, even though on biopsy there is no

evidence of these conditions. Typically, a patch of alopecia with no folliculitis is seen (Figure 3.33). In more severe cases, even with extensive alopecia, there is still no evidence of inflammation (Figure 3.34).

Morphea (localized scleroderma)

Morphea may affect the frontal scalp region when it is also known as a 'coup de sabre' lesion because it resembles the scar of a saber cut. It may be associated with underlying bone atrophy. The skin becomes white, smooth, shiny and attached to deeper structures. The active edge has a lilac discoloration (Figure 3.35) and the hair is shed to leave a scarring alopecia.

X-ray epilation leading to later alopecia

Diffuse scarring alopecia may occur in patients who have received X-ray treatment for conditions such as

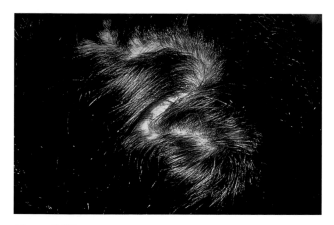

Figure 3.33

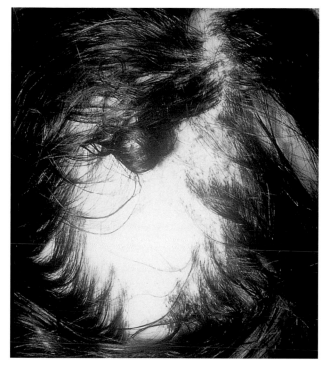

Figure 3.34

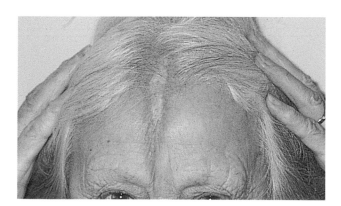

Figure 3.35

childhood scalp ringworm (Figure 3.36). Childhood X-ray epilation can not only cause scarring alopecia but also predispose to multiple basal and squamous cell carcinomas on the area of damaged skin (scar visible) (Figure 3.37).

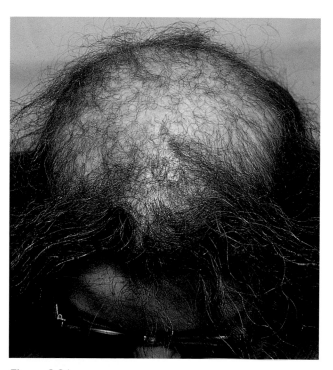

Figure 3.36

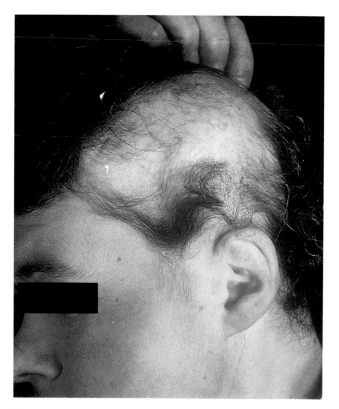

Figure 3.37

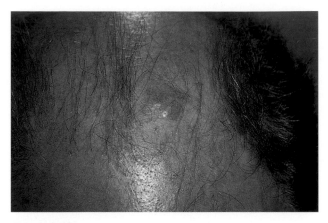

Figure 3.38

Figure 3.40

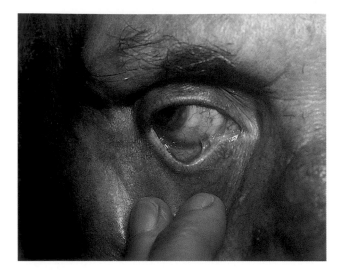

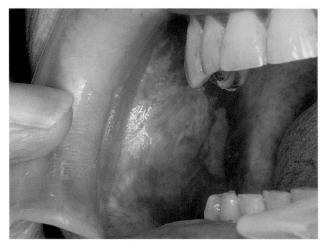

Figure 3.39

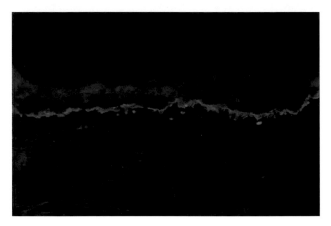

Figure 3.41

NON-SCARRING ALOPECIA

Androgenetic alopecia

Cicatricial pemphigoid

This autoimmune blistering disease causes inflammation and scarring of the skin and mucous membranes (especially eyes (Figure 3.38), mouth (Figure 3.39) and anogenital areas). When the scalp is affected, areas of inflammatory scarring alopecia occur, sometimes with blistering (Figure 3.40). Direct immunofluorescence performed on a skin biopsy from the patient shows linear deposition of IgG, and/or IgA and/or C3 along the basement membrane zone (Figure 3.41). Treatment with topical steroids often needs to be supplemented with oral steroids and other immunosuppressive agents. Despite treatment, blistering and scarring of the conjunctivae may lead to blindness.

Androgenetic alopecia (male pattern baldness, common baldness) is an extremely common condition, affecting both men and women. Following puberty, terminal hair follicles undergo miniaturization to become vellus-type follicles. This is associated with a shortening of the anagen phase of the hair cycle (see Chapter 1), an increased shedding of telogen hairs and subsequent hair loss.

Degrees of hair loss are classified on the Hamilton scale (Figure 3.42). Hair loss begins with bitemporal recession and thinning at the vertex, although the lateral and posterior hair follicles are usually spared (Figures 3.42–3.45). Women may also show a 'male' pattern of hair loss but more commonly show a 'Ludwig' pattern of hair loss (Figures 3.46 and 3.47), with diffuse thinning over the vault of the scalp (Figures 3.48 and 3.49). Hair loss following puberty

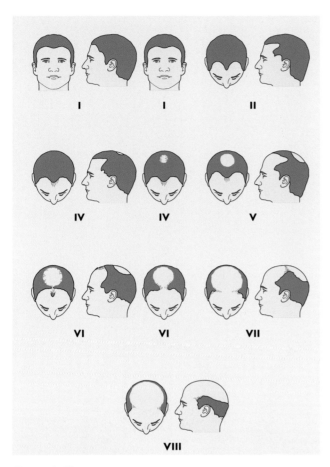

Figure 3.42

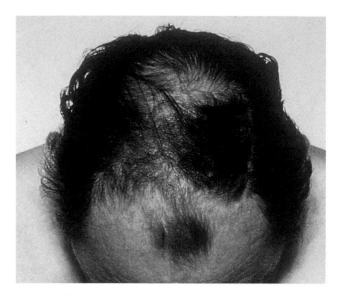

Figure 3.44

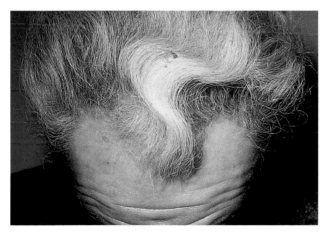

Figure 3.43

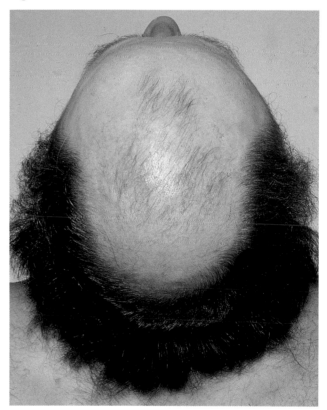

Figure 3.45

generally occurs more slowly in women than in men, but accelerates after the menopause, when Hamilton patterns of loss are more commonly seen. Androgenetic alopecia has been particularly studied in the stump-tailed macaque monkey where, interestingly, males and females are equally affected (Figure 3.50).

The pattern of inheritance of androgenetic alopecia remains unclear. Hair loss occurs owing to the effect of androgens on genetically sensitive follicle receptors. Follicles contain the enzyme 5α-reductase, which converts testosterone to dihydrotestosterone (DHT). Adult males who lack this enzyme have normal testosterone levels and reduced levels of DHT. They have sparse secondary sexual hair and do not develop androgenetic alopecia. There are two isoenzymes of 5α-reductase, of which type 2 seems to play an important role in androgenetic alopecia. A

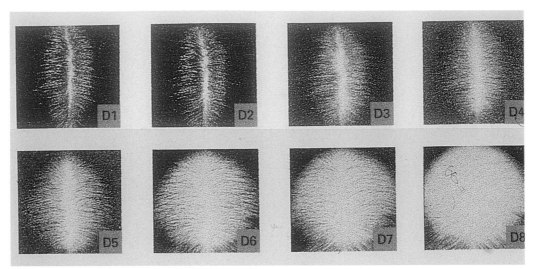

Figure 3.46

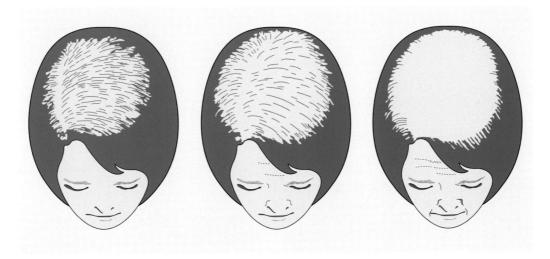

Figure 3.47

type-2 5α-reductase inhibitor (finasteride) has been safely used for many years to treat prostatic hypertrophy and is now being used therapeutically in men with androgenetic alopecia. Results of treatment for postmenopausal women have been disappointing. Other drug treatments include topical minoxidil and oral antiandrogens such as spironolactone and cyproterone acetate.

Telogen effluvium

Telogen effluvium is the temporary, diffuse shedding of hair, usually following physical or emotional stress (Figure 3.51). Normal hairs in the anagen growth phase are precipitated into the telogen phase, causing a fall of normal club-root hairs. Common stresses are febrile illness, major operations or blood loss. Hair loss usually occurs 6–16 weeks later and spontaneous regrowth usually occurs. Some degree of telogen effluvium follows normal pregnancy. Hormone levels during pregnancy inhibit hair follicles entering the catagen phase, causing anagen-phase hair numbers to increase. Following birth, follicles in which anagen has been prolonged rapidly enter catagen and subsequently telogen. Increased loss of hair usually begins a few weeks after birth and may continue for 4–6 months. No treatment is recommended, as recovery of normal hair density is spontaneous.

Endocrine causes of diffuse alopecia

Diffuse, non-scarring alopecia is a common symptom of many endocrine disorders. Hyperthyroidism and

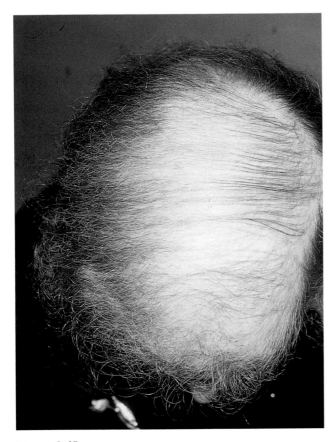

Figure 3.48

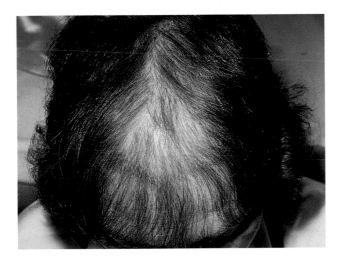

Figure 3.49

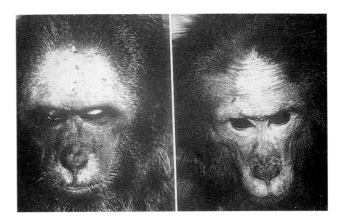

Figure 3.50

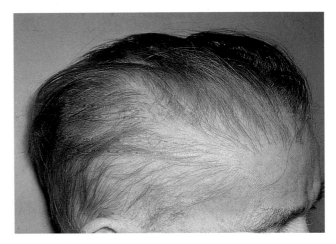

Figure 3.51

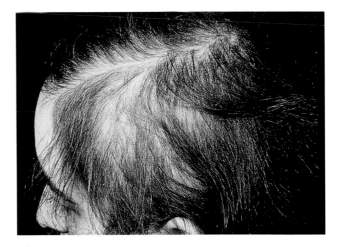

Figure 3.52

Drug causes of diffuse alopecia

particularly hypothyroidism can cause a diffuse alopecia. Thinning of the scalp and body hair may be the only clinical sign of hypothyroidism (Figure 3.52). Alopecia due to hypothyroidism usually improves with thyroxine replacement.

Hypopituitarism is associated with thinned or absent hair, and dry skin with a yellow hue. Hypoparathyroidism causes thinning and dryness of scalp hair.

Anticoagulants of all classes cause an increased shedding of hairs. This ceases spontaneously on cessation of the drug. The majority of tumor chemotherapy regimens cause a diffuse or total alopecia (Figure 3.53). Anagen follicles are shed acutely and prema-

33

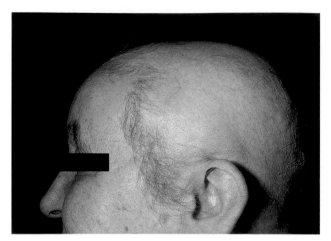

Figure 3.53

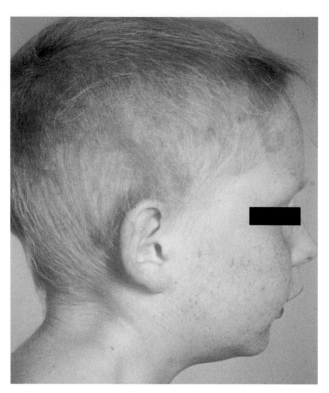

Figure 3.54

turely (anagen effluvium). Other hairs develop thinned shafts owing to inhibition of mitosis, and shedding is seen 4–6 days following the first chemotherapy dose. Techniques to cool the scalp during chemotherapy can help to minimize the affect on the follicles.

Systemic retinoids can cause a temporary kinking and thinning of the hair and consumption of large quantities of vitamin A can have a similar effect. There is some evidence that oral contraceptives occasionally cause temporary diffuse thinning of the hair, particularly 2–3 months after stopping the treatment as in pregnancy. β-Blockers, cimetidine, lithium carbonate and ibuprofen are among many other drugs implicated in causing diffuse hair thinning after prolonged treatment.

Metabolic and nutritional causes of alopecia

The two states of malnutrition, marasmus and kwashiorkor, both lead to hair becoming dry, brittle and thinned. Hair shafts can develop constrictions where they break easily, and black hairs can develop a red coloration. Anorexia nervosa can similarly be associated with hair thinning. Deficiencies of iron (Figure 3.54) and zinc (Figure 3.55) both cause diffuse alopecia. Zinc deficiency can additionally cause the cutaneous changes of dermatitis enteropathica (Figure 3.56).

Chronic diffuse alopecia

Chronic diffuse alopecia is the term used to describe either continuous or fluctuating diffuse hair loss, where the diagnosis is uncertain (Figure 3.57). It normally occurs in adults over 25 years of age, and presents more commonly in women. The underlying

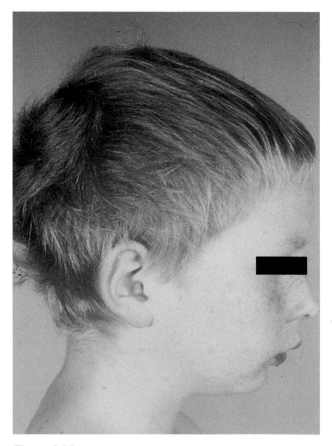

Figure 3.55

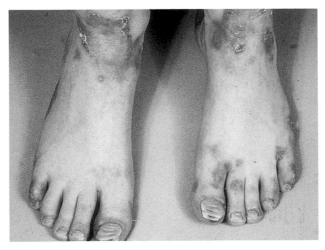

Figure 3.56

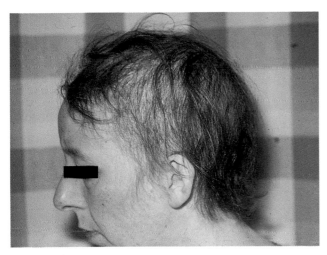

Figure 3.57

cause is often multifactorial. Mild androgenetic alopecia is often overlooked in women. The normal reduction of follicle numbers from the third decade onwards plays a role. The many causes of diffuse alopecia, including endocrine abnormalities, telogen effluvium, drugs and nutritional factors may be important. If no underlying cause can be found and the scalp and hair (both thickness and structure) are normal on examination, a diagnosis of dysmorphophobia should be considered. In this disorder, the patient remains convinced that her appearance is abnormal despite reassurance to the contrary.

REFERENCES

1. Labwohl M. New treatments for alopecia areata. *Lancet* 1997;349:222–3
2. Hordinsky MK. Alopecia areata. In Olsen EA, ed. *Disorders of Hair Growth.* New York: McGraw Hill, 1994
3. Messenger AG, Simpson NB. Alopecia areata. In Dawber RPR, ed. *Diseases of Hair and Scalp*, 3rd edn. Oxford: Blackwell Scientific Publications, 1997:338–69
4. Powell J, Dawber RPR, Gatter K. Folliculitis decalvans including tufted folliculitis – clinical, histological and therapeutic findings. *Br J Dermatol* 1999;140:328–33
5. Nayer M, Dawber RPR. Pseudopelade or lichen planus? *Br J Dermatol* 1993;129:374–6
6. Wilson CL, Burge SM, Dean D, *et al.* A clinicopathological study of scarring alopecia in chronic cutaneous lupus erythematosus. *Br J Dermatol* 1992;126:307–9
7. Albert RE, Omran AR. Follow up study of patients treated with X-ray epilation for tinea capitis. Population characteristics, post treatment illness and mortality experience. *Arch Environ Health* 1968;17:899–912
8. Kurzhals G, Stolz W, Maciejewski W, *et al.* Localised cicatricial pemphigoid of the scalp of the Brunsting–Perry type. *Arch Dermatol* 1995;131:580–4
9. Ludwig E. Classification of the types of androgenetic alopecia occurring in the female sex. *Br J Dermatol* 1977;97:247
10. Venning V, Dawber RPR. Patterned androgenetic alopecia. *J Am Acad Dermatol* 1988;18:1073
11. Rittmaster RS. Finasteride. *N Engl J Med* 1994;330:120
12. Tosti A, Camancho-Martinez F, Dawber R. Management of androgenetic alopecia. *J Eur Acad Dermatol Venereol* 1999;12:205–14
13. Eckert J, Church RE, Ebling FL, Munro DS. Hair loss in women. *Br J Dermatol* 1967;79:543
14. Skelton JB. Postpartum alopecia. *Arch Dermatol* 1966;94:125
15. Freinkel RK, Freinkel N. Hair growth and alopecia in hypothyroidism. *Arch Dermatol* 1972;106:349
16. Wexler D, Pace W. Acquired zinc deficiency disease of the skin. *Br J Dermatol* 1977;96:669

4

Hirsuties and hypertrichosis

HIRSUTIES

Hirsuties is defined as growth of terminal hairs under the influence of androgens in women, in areas when secondary sexual hair grows in men at puberty. An example is hair growth in the beard and moustache areas in a young woman (Figure 4.1), but chest, lower abdomen, back and limbs may also be affected. It has been estimated that 10% of women feel the need to remove unacceptable coarse facial hair growing after puberty. It is not unusual to see increased hair in the moustache area in a woman, with inflamed papules around hair follicles – a sign that electrolysis treatment has been performed (Figure 4.2). Increased facial hair in an adult Asian female (Figure 4.3) is hard to assess. Individual, genetic and racial variations in hair growth and in acceptance of it are great. There is no clear distinction between physiologic and pathologic hair

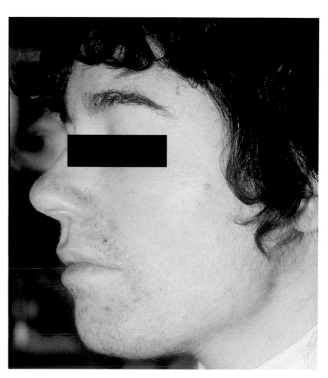

Figure 4.2

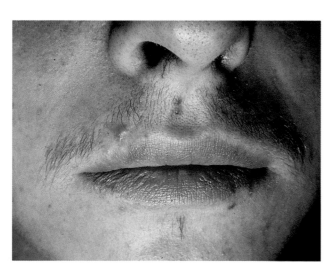

Figure 4.1

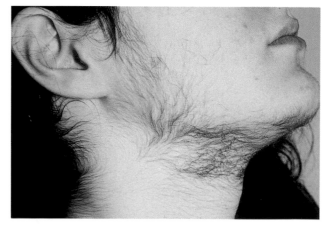

Figure 4.3

growth, since there is a spectrum of biologic variation.

Increased hair growth usually starts at puberty under the influence of androgens, and remains obvious through the potentially reproductive years. It may be associated with high androgen levels, acne and scanty or abnormal periods. It is not unusual, therefore, to see jaw-line and chin hair in a hirsute adult woman associated with signs of acne (Figure 4.4). Some degree of hirsutism after the menopause is very common (Figure 4.5).

HYPERTRICHOSIS

Hypertrichosis is defined as excessive growth of hair for a particular site and age of a patient (excluding androgen-induced hirsutism). 'Idiopathic' hypertrichosis may occur in any racial group, but is more common in Asians. Terminal hairs may be seen of the forehead (Figure 4.6), and eyebrows may be bushier than expected. This may be an isolated sign in an otherwise normal child, or may be part of one of a number of syndromes.

Hypertrichosis may be seen in association with congenital melanocytic nevi, as in Figure 4.7, which shows a well-circumscribed, pigmented lesion on the cheek which was present at birth. The hairs develop and become thicker and longer with age, and nodules may develop within the lesion. Such nevi may be large and extremely disfiguring, and carry a small but significant risk of developing malignant melanoma. Excision, in stages if necessary, may be advisable on cosmetic and prophylactic grounds where technically possible.

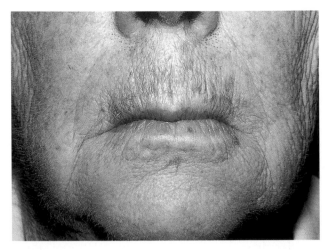

Figure 4.5

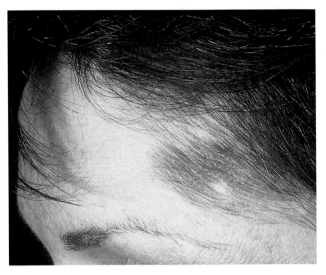

Figure 4.6

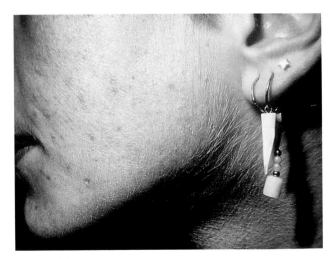

Figure 4.4

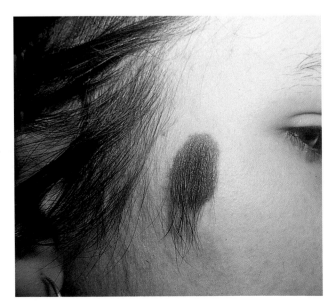

Figure 4.7

Hypertrichosis also occurs in Becker's nevus (Figure 4.8). This is a unilateral, segmental, acquired nevus, usually found on the upper back in young men. Gradually increasing pigmentation starts in childhood and coarse hairs develop at puberty (Figure 4.9). Acne vulgaris may be seen in the lesion, and it is possible that the affected area of skin has increased androgen receptor activity. Increased hair growth may also occur in a circumscribed 'nevoid' pattern with no other cutaneous change (no altered pigmentation). There may be single or multiple lesion(s). Localized increased hair growth is not unusual on the extensor surfaces of the arms ('elbow hypertrichosis') in children (Figure 4.10) and adults (Figure 4.11). Sometimes a circumscribed lumbosacral tuft of long silky hair overlying spinal dysraphism (failure of fusion) may be seen (see Figure 2.9). It is important in such cases to undertake full neurologic and radiologic investigation.

Another form of hypertrichosis, termed 'acquired lanuginosa', is a very rare disorder occurring in adults, where widespread lanugo hair develops on the face (Figure 4.12) and ear (Figure 4.13). This disorder is often associated with an internal malignancy.

Hypertrichosis may be drug-induced. Oral minoxidil prescribed for severe hypertension induces increased hair growth (including facial hair) (Figure 4.14) after a few weeks of treatment, and the hair is lost 2–3 months after stopping treatment. Topical minoxidil has similar, but more limited, effects. It is used to increase hair growth, but this is only sustained as long as the treatment continues. Cyclosporin, used as an immunosuppressive agent, may cause increased hair growth as seen here on the arms (Figure 4.15); it may also cause increased non-

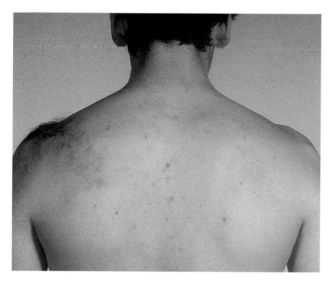

Figure 4.8

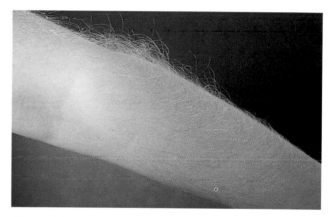

Figure 4.10

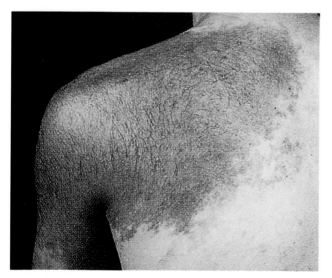

Figure 4.9

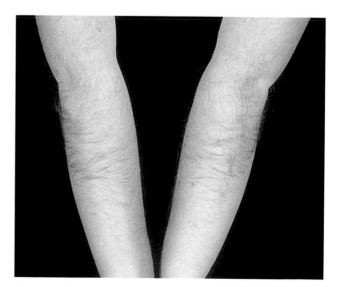

Figure 4.11

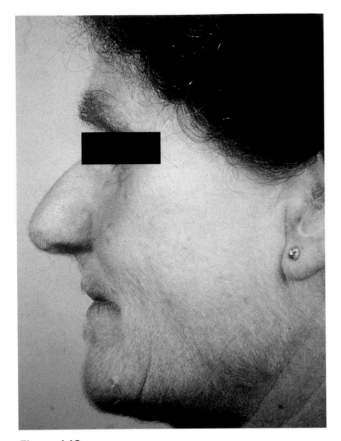

Figure 4.12

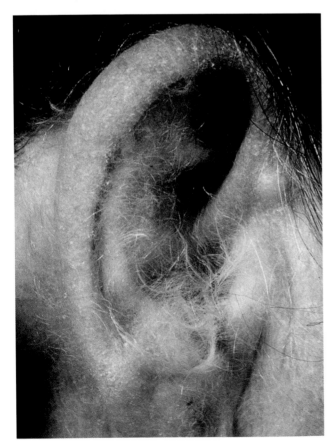

Figure 4.13

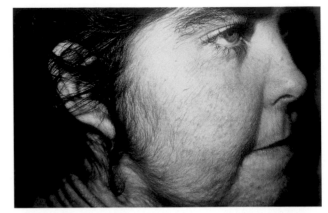

Figure 4.14

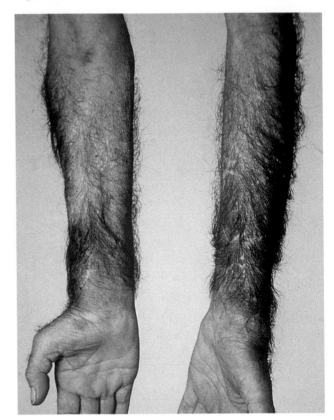

Figure 4.15

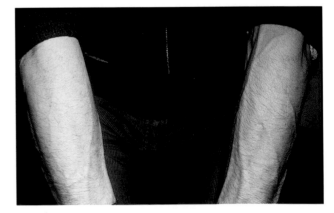

Figure 4.16

melanoma skin cancers. Another form of iatrogenic hypertrichosis may be seen when there is increased hair growth on a limb encased in plaster of Paris for a fracture. Figure 4.16 shows a patient's left arm which has been enclosed in plaster of Paris and which shows increased hair growth compared to the other arm.

REFERENCES

1. Barth JH. Hypertrichosis. In Dawber RPR, ed. *Diseases of Hair and Scalp*, 3rd edn. Oxford: Blackwell Scientific Publications, 1997:229–327

2. Barth JH, Wilkinson JD, Dawber RPR. Prepubertal hypertrichosis: normal or abnormal? *Arch Dis Child* 1988;63:666

3. Becker WS. Concurrent melanosis and hypertrichosis in the distribution of nevus unius lateris. *Arch Derm Syph* 1949;60:155

4. Simpson NB, Barth JH. Hair patterns: hirsuties and androgenetic alopecia. In Dawber RPR, ed. *Diseases of Hair and Scalp*, 3rd edn. Oxford: Blackwell Scientific Publications, 1997:67–122

5. Ewing JA, Rouse BA. Hirsutism, race and testosterone levels: comparison of east Asians and Euro-Americans. *Hum Biol* 1978;50:209

5

Disorders of the hair shaft

WEATHERING OF THE HAIR SHAFT

All hair fibers undergo some degree of breakdown of the cuticle (and possibly the cortex) from root to tip before being shed during the telogen or early anagen phase of the hair cycle. This is due to a combination of environmental (natural friction, wetting and ultraviolet radiation) and cosmetic factors such as combing, brushing, bleaching and permanent waving. Scalp hair, with its long anagen phase and length, is more susceptible than body hair.

Scanning electron micrographs (EM) of normal (unweathered) hair near to the root show closely apposed overlapping cuticular cells, which are also closely apposed to the underlying cortex (Figure 5.1). Further from the root in normal (weathered) hair, the cuticular 'scales' are slightly raised and have traumatized free margins (Figure 5.2). With increased weathering, there is progressive cuticle loss, fissuring and exposure of cortical cells (usually only seen near the tip) (Figure 5.3). Light microscopy (Figure 5.4) and scanning EM (Figure 5.5) of a weathered hair show loss of pigment, irregularly variable bore of the hair shaft and a transverse fissure in the cuticle, the ragged edges forming a 'node' or 'trichorrhexis nodosa', and, at the tip, the

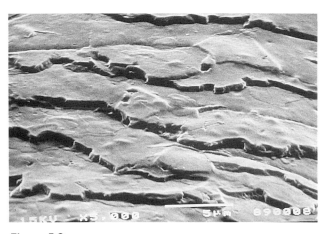

Figure 5.2

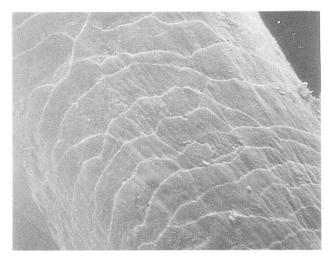

Figure 5.1

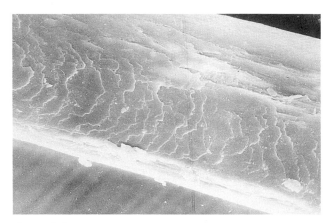

Figure 5.3

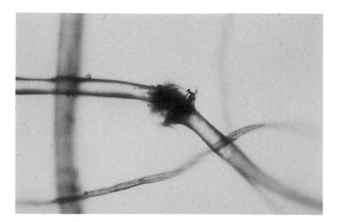

Figure 5.4

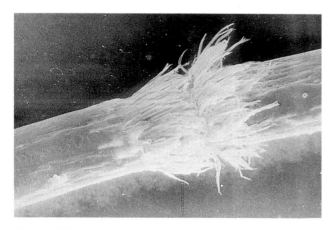

Figure 5.5

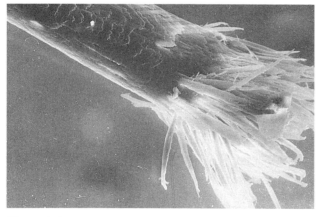

Figure 5.6

'brush tip' end of exposed cortical longitudinal cells (Figure 5.6).

STRUCTURAL DEFECTS OF HAIR LEADING TO INCREASED FRAGILITY

Any of the following defects of the hair shaft may present with patchy or diffuse alopecia. Although

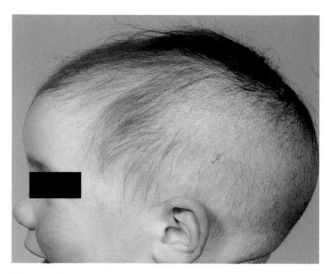

Figure 5.7

the structure of the hair shaft is unchangeable, it is possible to limit the changes in the hair by avoiding known causes of weathering.

Monilethrix ('necklace hair')

Monilethrix is an autosomal dominant condition in which the hair shaft is beaded and brittle and does not reach a normal length (Figure 5.7). It varies considerably in age of onset, severity and clinical course, owing to different genotypes or variable expressivity of the gene. In an adult patient, there may be short, broken scalp hairs of irregular length, and associated keratotic follicular papules (Figure 5.8), while a child may present with irregular severe hair loss. This may occur in the first few months of life, or be delayed until early adulthood. Occasionally, the disorder is revealed only after vigorous brushing. The beaded appearance of an affected hair in monilethrix can be seen on light microscopy (Figure 5.9) and with scanning EM (Figure 5.10).

The natural course of monilethrix varies, but there is a tendency for it to improve after puberty. Avoidance of trauma and cosmetic procedures is also helpful. Monilethrix-like beading may result from intermittent narrowing of the hair shaft due to bolus doses of cytotoxic chemotherapy (Figure 5.11) and there may be a prolonged narrowing of the hair shaft (Figure 5.12). When all hairs are affected with bolus treatment, the changes may be apparent over large areas of the scalp, the so-called 'flag sign'

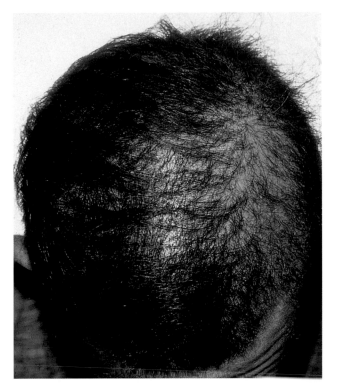

Figure 5.8

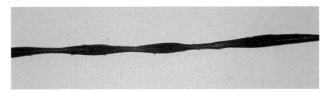

Figure 5.9

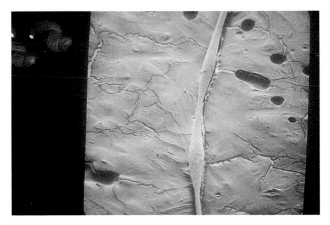

Figure 5.10

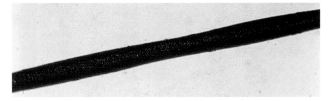

Figure 5.11

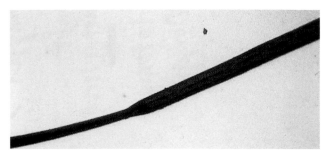

Figure 5.12

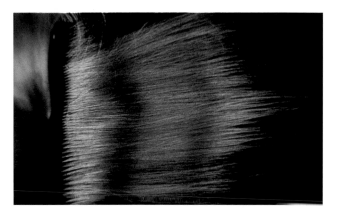

Figure 5.13

(Figure 5.13). Similar changes may occur with intermittent illness, the 'Pohl–Pinkus constriction'.

Pseudomonilethrix

A beaded appearance similar to that seen in monilethrix may be produced accidentally if hairs are pressed across each other during microscopic mounting. 'Pseudomonilethrix' may be seen in light micrographs (Figure 5.14) and EM (Figure 5.15) of normal hair.

Pili torti ('twisted hair')

In children with pili torti or twisted hair, the hair is normal at birth, but within months appears spangled, blond and unruly. Irregular breakages and weathering lead to variable thinning of the hair (Figure 5.16). This condition has an autosomal dominant inheritance, and may present from 3 months to 3 years or, occasionally, post-pubertally. Adults with pili torti have brittle hair which spangles in reflected light (Figure 5.17). Some length of hair growth may be achieved in some patients because it may be that not all hairs are affected (Figure 5.18), but, in others, only sparse stubble remains. Local inflammatory processes may also lead to focal irregular 'acquired'

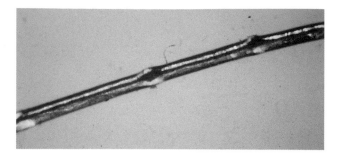

Figure 5.14

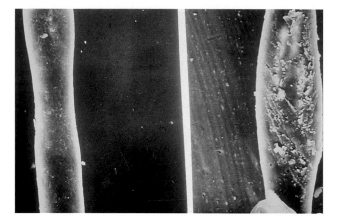

Figure 5.15

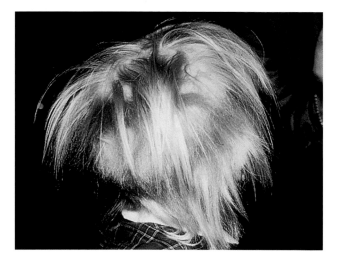

Figure 5.16

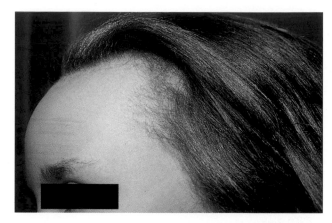

Figure 5.17

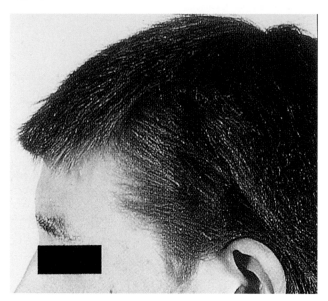

Figure 5.18

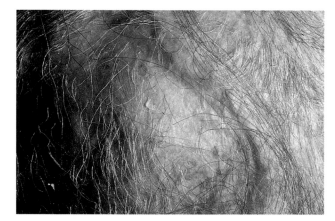

Figure 5.19

pili torti, shown here around the edges of patches of scarring alopecia (Figure 5.19). Light micrographs show the hairs to be flattened, and, at irregular intervals, completely rotated through 180° around their long axis (Figure 5.20). Scanning EM also shows the twisted hair shaft (Figure 5.21). This type of twisting may also be associated with a number of other shaft defects:

(1) Menkes' syndrome – light-colored, twisted hair seen in patients with an autosomal recessive hereditary defect of copper transport and ceruloplasmin;

(2) Hypohidrotic-ectodermal-dysplasia, in which twisted hairs are associated with characteristic facies and abnormalities of teeth and nails;

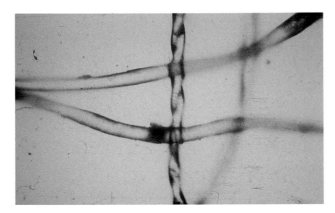

Figure 5.20

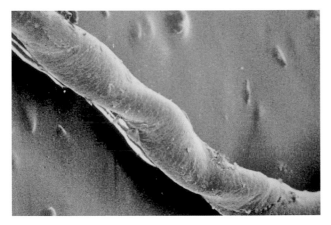

Figure 5.21

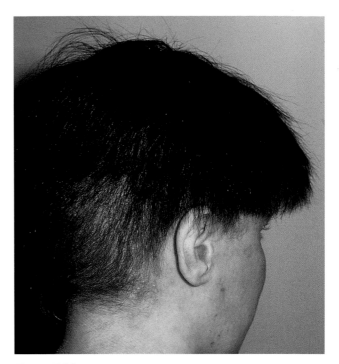

Figure 5.22

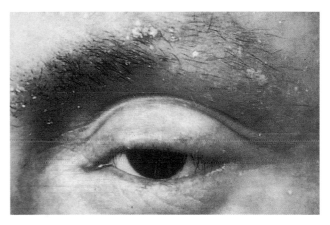

Figure 5.23

(3) Bjornstad's syndrome – twisted hair and sensorineural deafness;

(4) Bazex syndrome – twisted hair associated with basal cell carcinomas of the face and follicular atrophoderma;

(5) Trichothiodystrophy – see below.

Nethertons syndrome ('bamboo hair')

Netherton described characteristic 'bamboo node' changes in the hair associated with a red scaly dermatitis known as ichthyosis linearis circumflexa (ILC). Children with Netherton's syndrome may present with failure to thrive, or become acutely unwell in infancy with erythroderma, and 75% have associated atopy. Scalp hair is short, brittle, lusterless, sparse in patches (Figure 5.22) and rarely needs cutting. Eyebrows and facial hair are also sparse, short and dry (Figure 5.23). Lesions on the skin in Netherton's syndrome are erythematous, fine, dry and scaly, with a variably patterned serpiginous red border – ILC (Figure 5.24). Light microscopy reveals the pathognomonic 'bamboo nodes' (Figure 5.25).

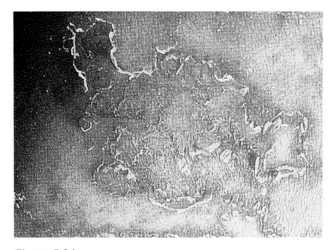

Figure 5.24

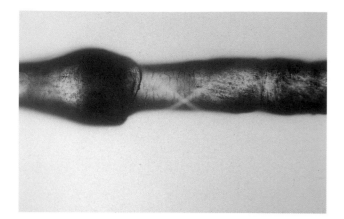

Figure 5.25

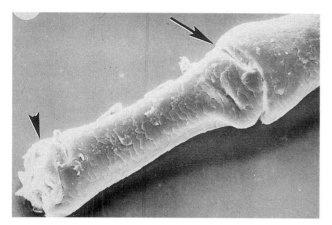

Figure 5.26

Scanning EM of affected hairs reveals 'trichorrhexis invaginata' (Figure 5.26). The nodes of trichorrhexis invaginata are a dilatation consisting of a bulbous hair end invaginating into a concave dilated proximal hair terminal. The only clue may be a ragged, cupped proximal hair end where the fragile node has fractured – 'golf tee hairs' (arrowhead); this is still diagnostic of Netherton's syndrome.

Trichothiodystrophy

Trichothiodystrophy is a term used to describe brittle hair with an abnormally low sulfur content, which weathers badly. The abnormality may be limited to the hair, or there may be associated features. These include ichthyosis, nail defects, mental retardation, growth retardation, decreased fertility, neutropenia and photosensitivity, and sometimes DNA repair defect. Typical presentation in a child could be ichthyosis, growth retardation and short brittle hair (Figure 5.27), but there is considerable variation in associated features. Polarized light

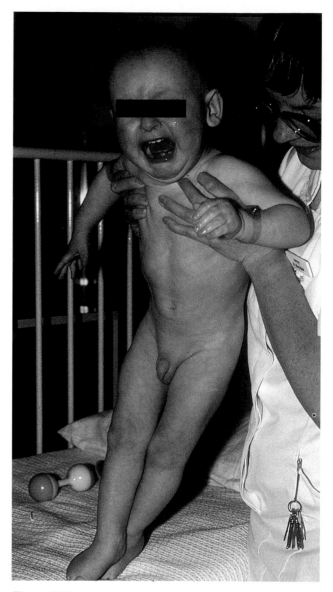

Figure 5.27

microscopy shows a banded appearance of hair from an affected patient. The abnormally weathered shaft is irregular, with cuticular cells patchily absent. Polarizing microscopy may reveal this as alternating bright and dark zones (Figure 5.28).

Scanning EM of hairs affected by trichothiodystrophy show abnormally weathered hair with clean breaks or 'trichoschisis fissures' (Figure 5.29), as well as partial breaks of the hair shafts forming 'trichorrhexis nodes' (Figure 5.30). The hairs are often flattened and ribbon-like (Figure 5.31). An electron micrograph (silver methenamine stain) from an affected patient (Figure 5.32), as compared to that from a normal patient (Figure 5.33), shows loss of silver staining in the exocuticle and cortex, and an

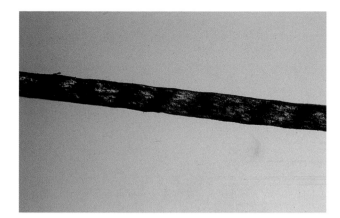

Figure 5.28

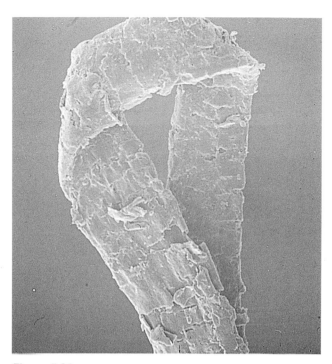

Figure 5.31

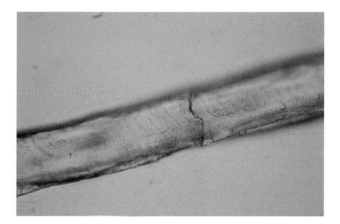

Figure 5.29

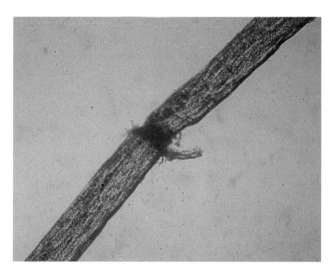

Figure 5.30

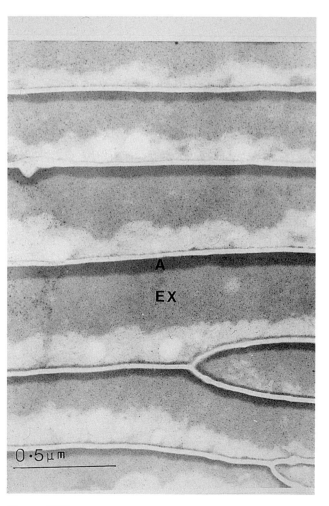

Figure 5.32

absent A layer. This illustrates the deficiency and disorganization of the incorporation of protein with a high sulfur content into the cortex and exocuticle, and absence of the layer of cuticle that normally has a homogeneous band of high-sulphur protein, which underlies the fragility of these hair fibers.

STRUCTURAL DEFECTS OF HAIR WITHOUT INCREASED FRAGILITY

Pili annulati ('ringed hair')

Pili annulati is frequently an incidental finding. The hair may appear slightly spangled, with alternating light and dark bands seen along each scalp hair (Figure 5.34) and plucked hair (Figure 5.35). The

abnormality lies in the light bands and is due to air spaces in the cortex. Hair reaches normal length and looks healthy. Light microscopy with transmitted light shows dark abnormal bands with a central pale area (Figure 5.36), while light microscopy with reflected light shows a dark central band (Figure 5.37). Scanning EM of transverse sections through

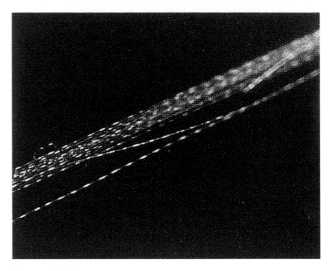

Figure 5.35

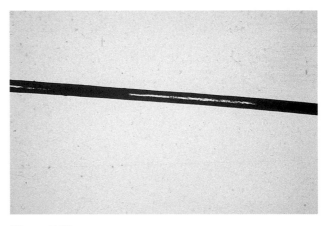

Figure 5.36

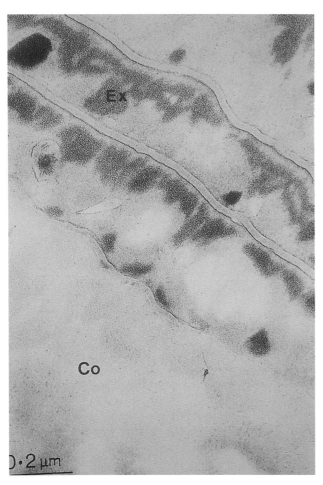

Figure 5.33

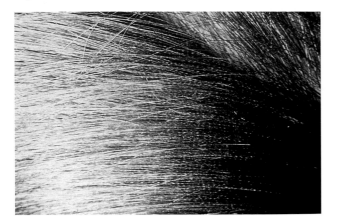

Figure 5.34

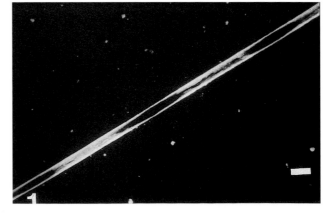

Figure 5.37

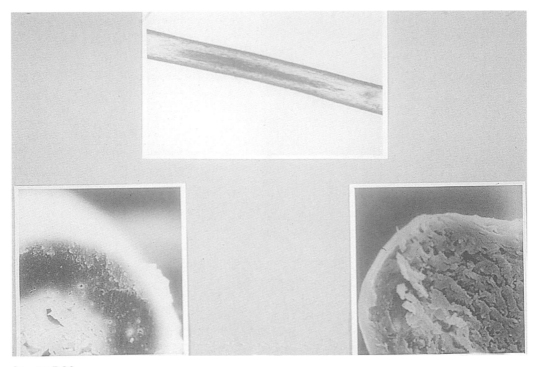

Figure 5.38

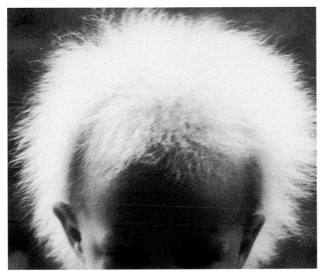

Figure 5.39

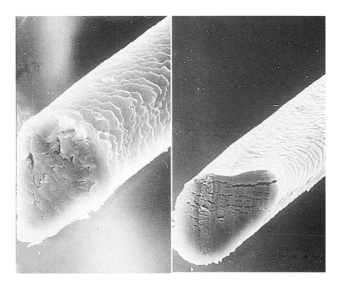

Figure 5.40

the abnormal band of an affected hair in pili annulati shows diffuse irregular spaces throughout the cortex (Figure 5.38), but, through a 'normal band' of an affected hair shows an outer ring of dense compact cortex and an organized, fenestrated central medulla.

Cheveux incoiffables

Cheveux incoiffables (uncombable hair syndrome, spun glass hair) is a fixed abnormality in the hair shaft that becomes obvious when the terminal hair grows in the first few years of life. The scalp hair has a wild disorderly appearance (Figure 5.39), although eyebrows and eyelashes are normal. The hair may reach normal length and the appearance often improves during childhood, although the structural abnormality persists. On scanning EM of an affected hair, a longitudinal canalicular gutter may be seen along the hair shaft (Figure 5.40), and the cross-section of the hair shaft is characteristically triangular or heart-shaped.

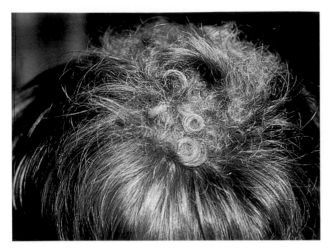

Figure 5.41

Woolly hair nevus

A woolly hair nevus is a congenital focal growth of abnormally crimped or curled hair, in the midst of normal scalp hair (Figure 5.41).

REFERENCES

1. Dawber RPR, Van Neste D. *Hair and Scalp Disorders: Common Presenting Signs, Differential Diagnosis and Treatment*. London: Martin Dunitz, 1995

2. Garcia ML, Epps JH, Yare RS. Normal cuticle wear patterns in human hair. *J Soc Cosm Chem* 1978;29:155

3. de Berker DAR, Dawber RPR. Monilethrix: clinical and microscopic findings in 21 cases. *Br J Dermatol* 1991;125:24

4. Netherton EW. A unique case of trichorrhexis nodosa, 'Bamboo hairs'. *Arch Dermatol* 1958;78:483–7

5. Judge MR, Morgan G, Harper JL. A clinical and immunological study of Netherton's syndrome. *Br J Dermatol* 1994;131:615–19

6. Van Neste DJJ, Gillespie JM, Marshall RC, *et al.* Morphological and biochemical characteristics of trichothiodystrophy variant hair are maintained after grafting of scalp specimens onto nude mice. *Br J Dermatol* 1993;128:384

7. Venning V, Dawber RPR, Ferguson DJP, *et al.* Weathering of hair in trichothiodystrophy. *Br J Dermatol* 1986;114:591

8. Mallon E, Dawber RPR, de Berker DAR, *et al.* Cheveux incoiffables – diagnostic, clinical and hair microscopic findings, and pathogenic studies. *Br J Dermatol* 1994;131:608–14

9. Whiting DA. Structural abnormalities of the hair shaft. *J Am Acad Dermatol* 1987;15:1

6

Infections and infestations of the hair and scalp

FUNGAL INFECTIONS

Tinea capitis

Tinea capitis (ringworm of the scalp) is caused by invasion of the hair shaft by a dermatophyte fungus. Dermatophytes belong to one of three groups, zoophilic, anthropophilic or geophilic, depending on their common habitat (animal, plant or soil). They are also divided into three genera, *Microsporum*, *Trichophyton* and *Epidermophyton*. The most common species involved vary over time and between different regions and countries. *Microsporum* and *Trichophyton* genera are both able to invade hair. *M. canis* and *M. audouini* are common infections in Europe, while *T. tonsurans* has become very common in the USA and is increasingly seen in the UK.

Scalp ringworm can cause alopecia, scaling, inflammation, scalp pustulation and breakage of hair. The clinical features vary depending on the type of infection and host response to it. Anthropophilic infections generally cause minor scaling and erythema (Figure 6.1). Zoophilic infections tend to stimulate a strong host response, which may result in the formation of a boggy inflammatory mass known as a kerion (Figure 6:2); this is sometimes mistaken for a more sinister tumor and treated inappropriately.

Dermatophytes invade hair in two different ways: ectothrix infection, where hyphae emerge through the hair surface and form masses predominantly on the external surface of the hair, and endothrix infection, where hyphae form spores which remain within the hair cortex. Ectothrix fungi, such as *M. canis* and *T. mentagrophytes*, cause hair to become dull and lusterless and to break off a few millimeters from the scalp. Endothrix fungi, such as *T. tonsurans*, cause more damage to the hair shaft, with hairs breaking off at the scalp surface. This can cause a 'black dot' appearance. *Microsporum* and *T. schoenleinii* infections often emit a green fluorescence under Wood's light (ultraviolet light passed through 9% nickel oxide glass) in the dark (Figure 6.3). Diagnosis is confirmed by microscopy and culture of hairs plucked from the affected area.

The standard treatment for tinea capitis is griseofulvin at a daily dose of 500–1000 mg for adults and 10 mg/kg for children, over 6–8 weeks. Kerion should additionally be treated with potent topical steroids to help reduce inflammation and limit scarring. Occasionally, systemic steroids may be necessary. Anthropophilic infections can be spread easily and affected children should probably be kept at home. Zoophilic fungi are much less infectious and affected children should be allowed to go to school. Other oral antifungals such as terbinafine may be used.

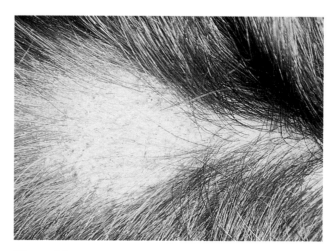

Figure 6.1

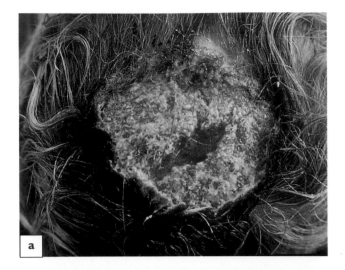

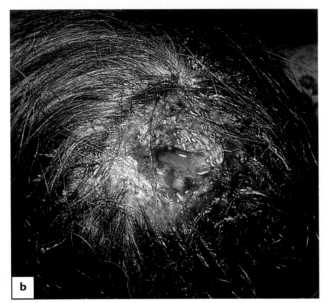

Figure 6.2

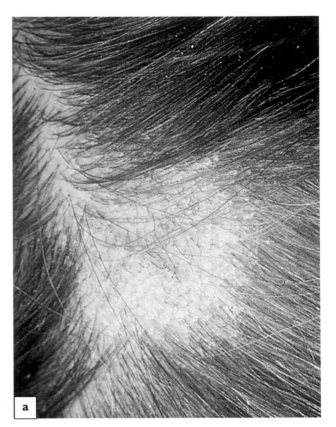

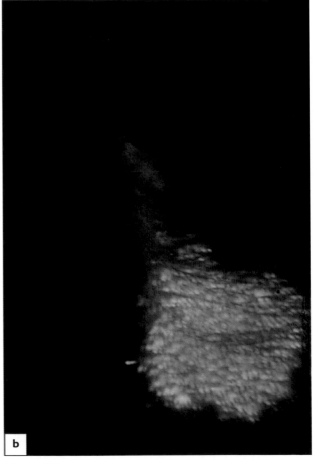

Figure 6.3

Favus

Favus is a type of chronic endothrix infection caused by *T. schoenleinii* in which the hair shaft is not weakened (Figure 6.4a). Hyphae grow down the hair shaft and cause the development of cup-shaped, yellow crusts around the hair follicle orifices called 'scutula' (Figure 6.4b).

Ringworm of the beard

Dermatophyte infection of the beard area (tinea barbae) can cause inflammation and pustulation (Figure 6.5). Zoophilic fungi are the most common causative species. Treatment should be with oral antifungal drugs with addition of topical steroids to reduce inflammation.

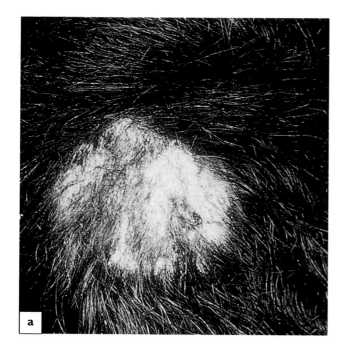

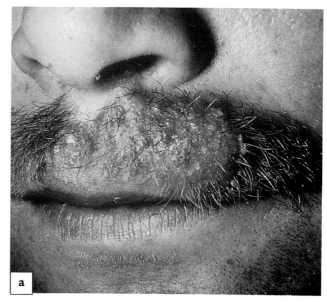

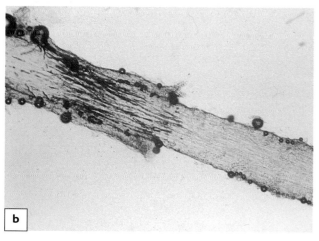

Figure 6.4

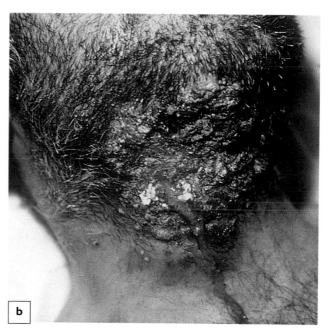

Figure 6.5

Black piedra

Black piedra is an infection of hair by the ascomycete fungus *Piedraia hortai*. It occurs endemically in the tropical areas of South and Central America and Malaysia. Affected hairs develop black, hard, nodules which are firmly adherent to the hair shaft (Figure 6.6).

White piedra

This is a rare infection of hair by the fungus *Trichosporon cutaneum* (also known as *T. Beigelii*). It forms white, soft, nodules on the hair shaft (Figure 6.7). Hair at any body site can be affected, but the genital region is most commonly affected.

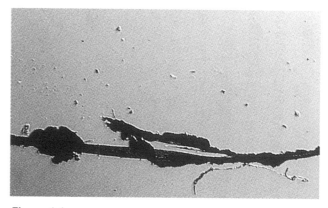

Figure 6.6

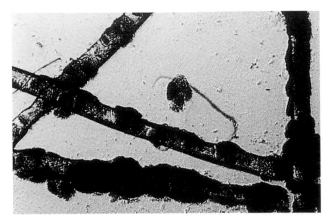

Figure 6.7

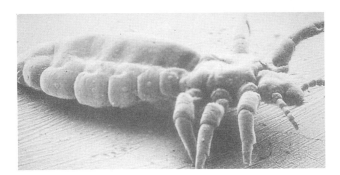

Figure 6.8

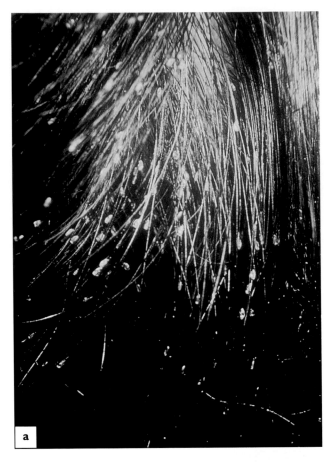

a

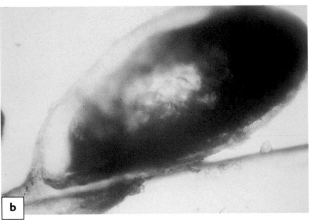

b

Figure 6.9

INFESTATIONS

Pediculosis capitis

Pediculosis capitis (infestation by *Pediculus humanus capitis*, or head lice) is a common infestation of the scalp, particularly amongst school-age children. Lice do not fly or jump, but can run quickly. Transmission occurs via close contact or via shared brushes/combs. Infestation causes intense itching of the scalp and frequently the development of itchy, urticated papules on the back of the neck. Adult lice (Figure 6.8) may be seen moving with the naked eye. Eggs (nits) adhere firmly to the hair shaft and can therefore be easily distinguished from dandruff both with the naked eye and microscopically (Figure 6.9). Prolonged infestation can lead to secondary bacterial infection of the scalp with associated lymphadenopathy. Standard treatments include the use of shampoos and lotions containing insecticides such as malathion, carboryl or permethrin, in conjunction with combing to physically remove the eggs, but resistance to these insecticides is now increasing. The cyclical use of intensive combing of the hair is recommended, aided by copious hair conditioner to reduce friction and remove adult lice before further

eggs are laid. All family members and close contacts should be offered treatment at the same time to prevent reinfection.

Pediculosis pubis

Pediculosis pubis (infestation by *Phthirius pubis*, the crab or pubic louse, Figure 6.10) is most commonly sexually transmitted but can be contracted via infested clothing. The crab louse can infest all sites of body hair, including eyebrows and lashes, apart from the scalp. Treatment is usually with gamma benzene hexachloride applied topically to all affected areas and washed off 24 h later.

Ticks

Ticks are blood-sucking ectoparasites which attach firmly to the skin (Figure 6.11). They may cause a localized eczematous eruption or urticaria. Some species occasionally act as vectors for diseases such as Lyme disease, tick typhus or Rocky Mountain spotted fever. Simply scraping off a tick from the skin will leave the mouth-parts *in situ*. They should be removed with forceps, gripped tightly at the entry point into the skin.

BACTERIAL INFECTIONS

Trichomycosis axillaris

Trichomycosis axillaris (sticky armpit disease) is a superficial aerobic *Corynebacterium* infection of axil-

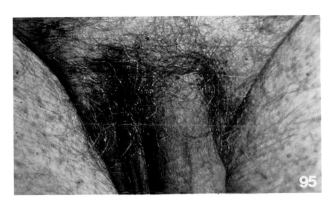

Figure 6.10

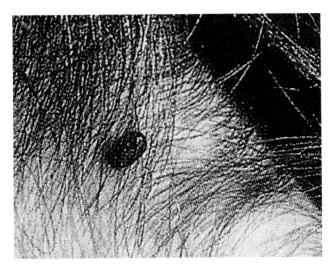

Figure 6.11

lary or occasionally pubic hair. Firmly adherent concretions form on the hairs, which may be yellow, red or black (Figure 6.12). Sweat may be colored and cause staining of clothes.

Lupus vulgaris

Lupus vulgaris is one form of cutaneous tuberculosis where reddish-brown plaques are formed with a classical 'apple-jelly' nodule appearance at the edge. The majority (80%) of European cases occur on the head and neck. Single plaques may occur or disease can be more extensive (Figure 6.13). Diagnosis can be confirmed from histological examination and culture of a skin biopsy. Treatment should be with standard antituberculous therapy.

VIRAL INFECTIONS

Viral warts

Viral warts are caused by several types of human papilloma virus. Warts affecting the scalp are often

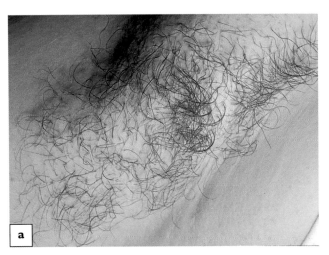

a

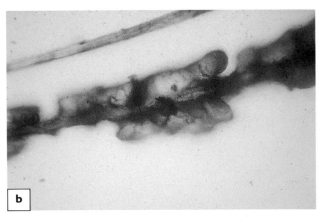

b

Figure 6.12

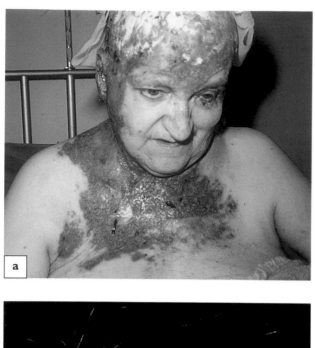

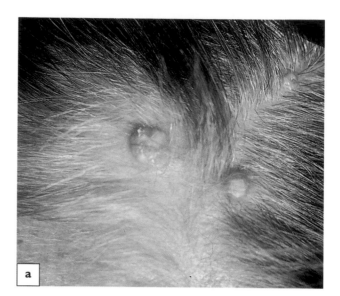

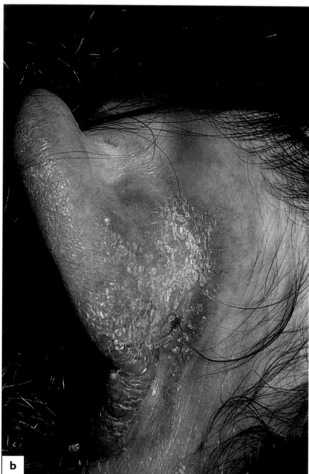

Figure 6.13

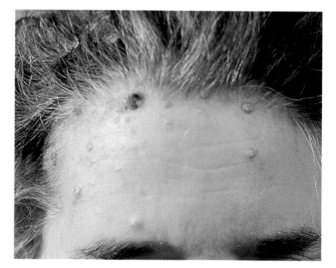

Figure 6.14

hyperkeratotic and filiform (Figure 6.14). They can be troublesome when combing the hair. Warts may be left alone to clear spontaneously. Treatment options otherwise include cryotherapy, curettage and cautery or topical salicylic acid preparations.

Figure 6.15

Molluscum contagiosum

Molluscum contagiosum is caused by a pox virus. Characteristic umbilicated pearly pink papules with a keratotic centre are seen commonly on the trunk and limbs of children and young adults with this condition (Figure 6.15). However, in immunosuppressed individuals, molluscum contagiosum may be found at any age and may affect the face and scalp.

REFERENCES

1. Elewski BE, Hazen PG. The superficial mycoses and the dermatophytes. *J Am Acad Dermatol* 1988;21:655

2. Mills CM, Philpot CM. Tinea capitis in S. Wales: observation of change in causative fungi. *Clin Exp Dermatol* 1994;19:473

3. Hay RJ, ed. *Fungi and Skin Disease*. London: Gower Medical Publishing, 1993

4. Hakendorf AJ, Donald GF, Linn HW. Favus. *Aust J Dermatol* 1965;8:22

5. Drake LA, Dinehart S, Farmer ER. Guidelines for the care of superficial mycotic infections of the skin: piedra. *J Am Acad Dermatol* 1996;94:122

6. Fisher I, Morton RS. *Phthirius pubis* infestation. *Br J Vener Dis* 1970;46:326

7. Wilson C, Dawber RPR. Trichomycosis axillaris – a different view. *J Am Acad Dermatol* 1989;21:325

8. Reveri M, Krishnamurthy C. Gonococcal scalp abscess. *J Pediatr* 1979;94:819

7

Scalp dermatoses

Many skin diseases may affect the scalp and hair.

SEBORRHEIC DERMATITIS OF THE SCALP

Seborrheic dermatitis in its mildest form causes pityriasis capitis or 'dandruff' of the scalp. There is no inflammation, although the patient may complain their scalp is itchy. The main symptom and finding is a fine scaling of the scalp (Figure 7.1), which may be associated with itchy red scaly lesions at the margins of the scalp (Figure 7.2) and the sides of the nose and anterior chest. Yeast-like organisms (*Pityrosporum ovale*) can be found. The increased scaling may be seen as 'pseudo nits', peripilar keratin casts which are formed in the hair follicle infundibulum, possibly by the internal root sheath's failing to desquamate normally from the follicular opening and becoming wrapped around the hairs (Figure 7.3). These may be seen more clearly in a light micrograph (Figure 7.4) or electron micrograph (Figure 7.5), in which the peripilar keratin cast can be seen to be not attached to the underlying hair, but surrounding it.

PSORIASIS OF THE SCALP

Psoriasis is an inflammatory dermatosis affecting 2% of the population of Western countries. The exact cause is unknown, but there is a genetic predisposition to the development of the disease. Lesions may be precipitated by infections, trauma and stress. It commonly affects the scalp (and may affect only the scalp) causing severe scaling and peripilar keratin casts (Figure 7.6). Red, scaly, well-demarcated lesions are often visible at the hair margin, but also occur on the hair-bearing areas of the scalp (Figure

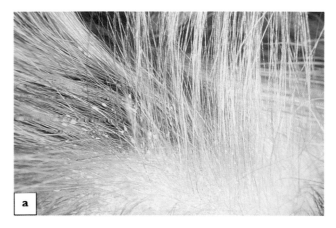

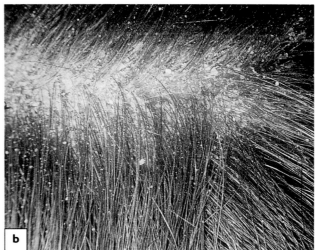

Figure 7.1

7.7). They are thick and palpable, and vary from one or two plaques to a whole sheet covering the entire surface of the scalp. Nail lesions are frequent and typical in psoriasis, and are useful diagnostic clues if skin lesions are few, or the patient has isolated scalp lesions. The two characteristic changes are pitting of the nail, where the pits may be large and irregular,

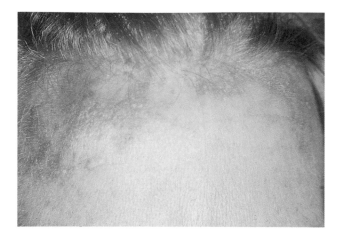

Figure 7.2

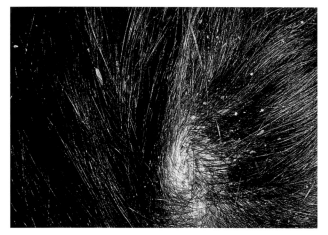

Figure 7.3

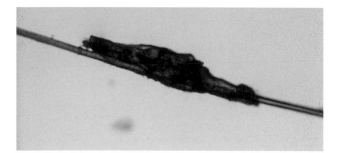

Figure 7.4

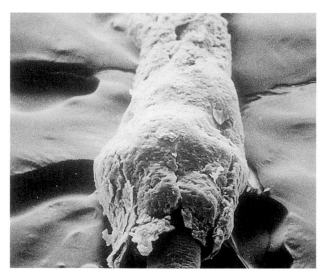

Figure 7.5

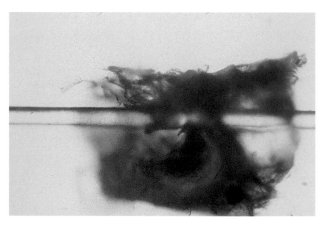

Figure 7.6

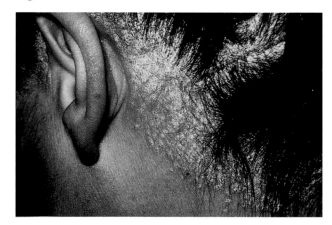

Figure 7.7

and 'onycholysis' or lifting of the nail plate, which may lead to discoloration of the nail (Figure 7.8).

PITYRIASIS AMIANTACEA

Psoriatic scale may occasionally become very thick indeed, and stick in large chunks to the proximal ends of groups of hairs (Figure 7.9). This may also be seen in other disorders of the scalp causing increased scaling, such as atopic eczema and fungal infections. There may also be temporary hair loss associated with severe scalp psoriasis.

Treatment is by means of shampoos and gels containing emollients, tar, keratolytics (e.g. Unguentum Cocois Co. containing tar and salicylic

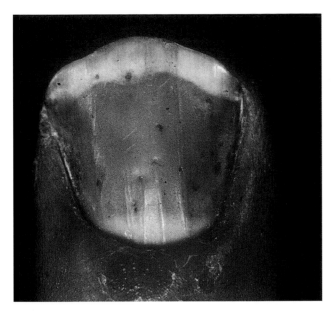

Figure 7.8

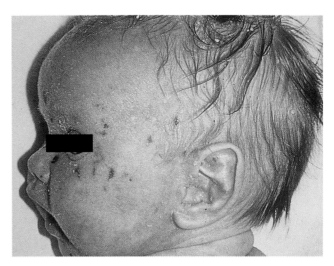

Figure 7.10

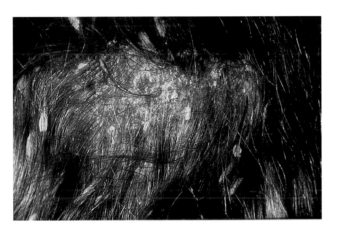

Figure 7.9

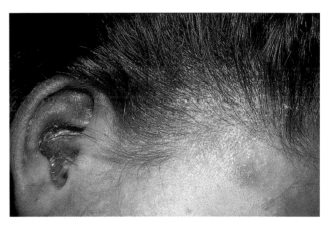

Figure 7.11

acid is massaged in at night and washed out the following morning). Topical steroid lotions may also be useful.

ATOPIC DERMATITIS

Atopy implies a genetic predisposition to develop eczema, asthma and hay fever, commonly presenting in infancy and childhood. Eczema and dermatitis are synonymous, and cause an inflammatory reaction pattern in the skin that is itchy, and may show erythema, edema, papules, vesicles and exudation, as seen on the face and scalp of the infant in Figure 7.10. Atopic dermatitis may also affect adults, for example on the ear and scalp margin (Figure 7.11). Treatments include emollients, topical steroid preparations, antibiotics for secondary infections (which

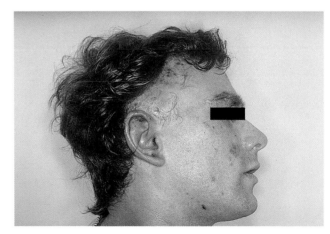

Figure 7.12

are common), and a sympathetic explanation of the nature of the disorder. The pruritus of atopic dermatitis leads to chronic rubbing and scratching, which may cause thickening or 'lichenification' of the skin, and loss of hair of the scalp (Figure 7.12) or eyebrow. Scratching the pruritic areas may also lead to erosions of skin and a subsequent increased risk of secondary infection (Figure 7.13).

ALLERGIC CONTACT DERMATITIS

Allergic contact dermatitis develops as a delayed hypersensitivity reaction to an external allergen, usually after repeated exposure, but rarely after one

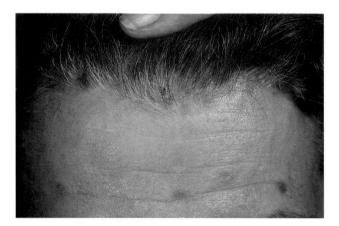

Figure 7.13

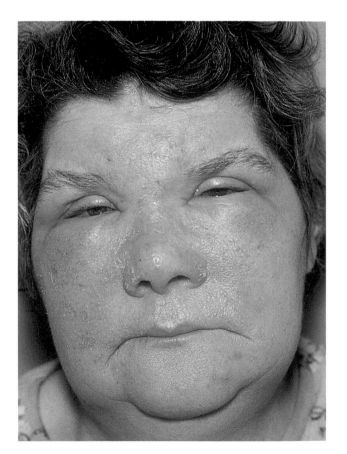

Figure 7.14

exposure. The scalp may have only minimal inflammation while the face and neck are severely affected. Allergy may develop suddenly, after years of exposure to the allergen without problems. Paraphenylenediamine hair dye is a common allergen, and may cause dermatitis at the hair margins, eyelids and face (Figure 7.14; see also Figure 9.2), but usually causes very little problem on the scalp itself.

Nail varnish is another common sensitiser, and the resulting dermatitis is often seen around the hair margins and neck where the fingers have touched the skin. Similarly, glues and dyes used in hats may lead to 'hatband dermatitis' around the forehead (Figure 7.15). Patch testing elicits a delayed hypersensitivity response 48–72 h after contact, and helps reach a diagnosis if interpreted in the context of the patient's presenting problem.

LICHEN SIMPLEX CHRONICUS

Irritation leads to constant rubbing and scratching which causes thickening or 'lichenification' of the skin. The 'itch–scratch cycle' is hard to break, and long-standing plaques develop on the skin, one typical site being the anterior (Figure 7.16) or posterior hair margin (lichen nuchae). It may also occur on the shins, forearms or vulval and perianal areas. Treatment with potent topical steroids under occlusion may help, but the problem tends to recur.

DARIER'S DISEASE

Darier's disease (keratosis follicularis) is an autosomal dominant inherited disease causing abnormal

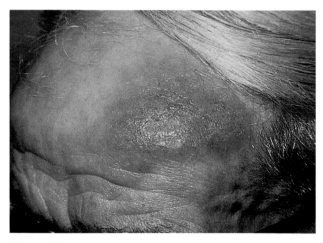

Figure 7.15

keratinization. Pigmented follicular keratotic papules develop over the face and neck (Figure 7.17), usually first appearing in adolescence. Typical lesions are also seen in the groin (Figure 7.18) and axillae, and central chest and back. The keratotic warty-looking lesions may become secondarily infected and malodorous, and may cause considerable hair loss.

Systemic retinoids are useful in controlling symptoms in severely affected patients. The nail changes are pathognomonic – longitudinal white and pink bands, with V-shaped notches at the free end of the nail occurring at the end of the band (Figure 7.19).

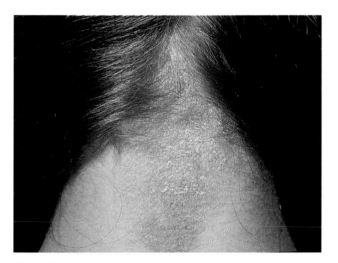

Figure 7.16

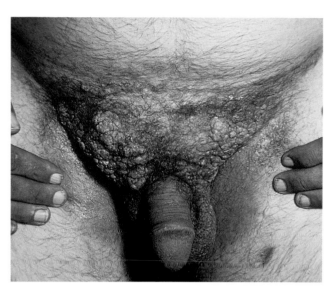

Figure 7.18

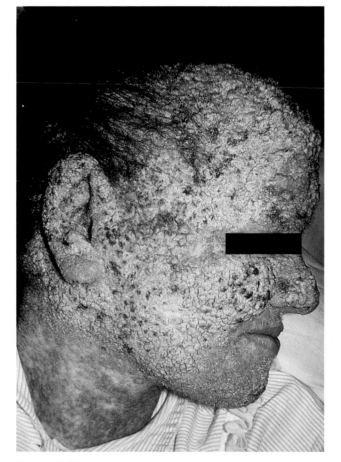

Figure 7.17

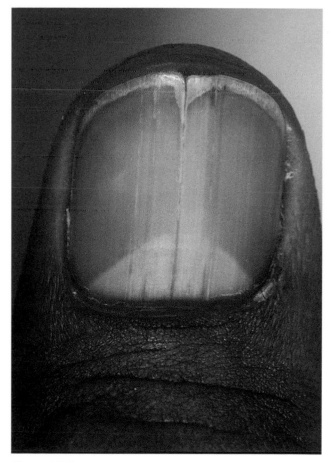

Figure 7.19

EROSIVE PUSTULAR DERMATOSIS OF THE SCALP

This is usually seen in elderly patients, sometimes precipitated by trauma, most often in sun-damaged skin with associated solar keratoses. An area of the scalp becomes inflamed and edematous with pustules and crusting (Figure 7.20). It may resemble a developing malignancy (Figure 7.21), but, if diagnosed correctly and treated with potent topical steroids, it resolves promptly to reveal normal (though still sun-damaged) skin.

PITYRIASIS RUBRA PILARIS

In this rare disorder, reddish/orange follicular keratotic lesions may be localized or generalized. If localized, there are well-demarcated scaly plaques (Figure

7.22). If pityriasis rubra pilaris becomes generalized, there are usually characteristic 'islands of sparing' but exfoliative dermatitis may occur. There is usually an associated thickening of the palmar and plantar skin, with nail dystrophy.

FOLLICULAR MUCINOSIS

This presents with infiltrated, erythematous plaques with follicular involvement and hair loss (Figure 7.23). It may present in childhood when it is usually benign, but in adults it may be associated with mycosis fungoides (cutaneous T-cell lymphoma) (Figure 7.24). Skin manifestations are the first and often the only expression of the disease.

SARCOIDOSIS

This is a multi-system granulomatous disorder, the cause of which remains unknown. One of the patterns of skin involvement is papules, nodules and

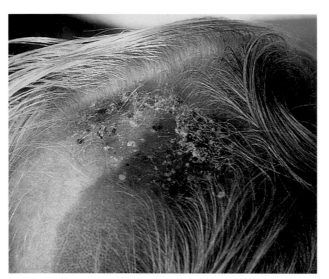

Figure 7.20

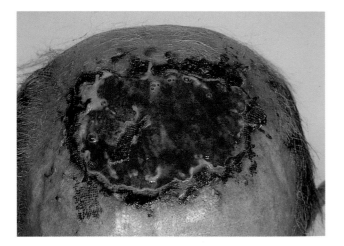

Figure 7.21

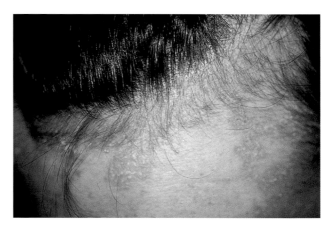

Figure 7.22

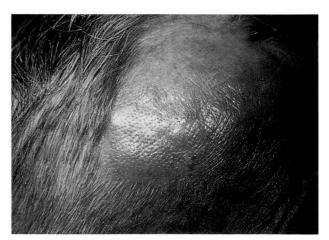

Figure 7.23

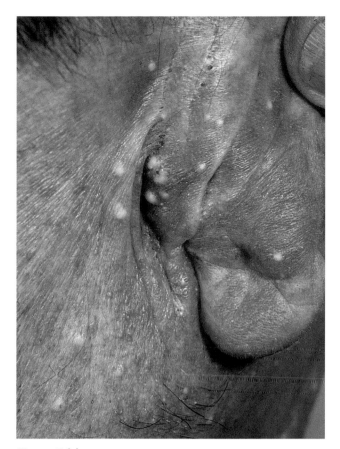

Figure 7.24

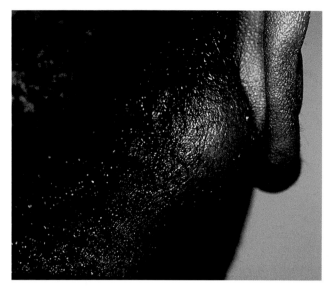

Figure 7.26

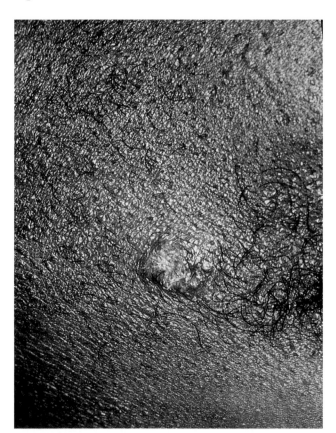

Figure 7.25

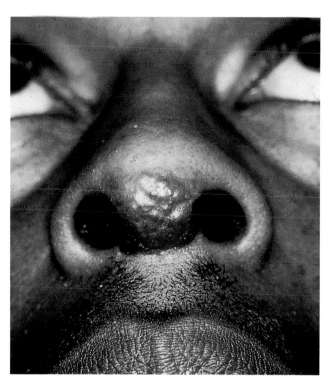

Figure 7.27

plaques that may cause alopecia in the scalp and beard area (Figure 7.25), often with associated lymphadenopathy, as seen here in the postauricular node (Figure 7.26). It may also cause erythema nodosum, swelling and discoloration of the ears and nose (Figure 7.27), and localization to old scar tissue. Treatment involves systemic steroids, especially if there is serious internal involvement, e.g. chest or liver disease.

DERMATOMYOSITIS

Dermatomyositis is an autoimmune disease affecting skin and muscle. If it presents in childhood, vasculitis and calcinosis and considerable scarring may occur with resulting alopecia. In the elderly, it may be associated with malignancy. Diffuse alopecia occurs in up to 15% of patients in the acute stage, but complete regrowth of hair is usual. In chronic disease, inflammatory lesions become atrophic, and, on hair-bearing areas, cicatricial alopecia results, seen with other characteristic skin changes including violaceous or 'heliotrope' discoloration of the eyelids and face (Figure 7.28), and linearly on the dorsal aspect of the fingers with nail-fold telangiectasia (Figure 7.29). The mainstay of treatment is oral steroids, combined with other immunosuppressants such as azathioprine, methotrexate and cyclophosphamide. Physiotherapy is very important if there is significant muscle involvement.

HISTIOCYTOSIS

Owing to the proliferation of Langerhans cells, histiocytosis may cause generalized severe diseases (Hand–Schuller–Christian disease, Letterer–Siwe disease, eosinophilic granuloma). Lesions on the scalp appear erythematous and indurated with a scaly surface (Figure 7.30), and a biopsy will differentiate them from seborrhoeic dermatitis or folliculitis.

ACNE KELOIDALIS NUCHAE

Acne keloidalis nuchae (folliculitis keloidalis) is a specific pattern of folliculitis most commonly seen in black men. Firm papules and pustules develop in a follicular pattern, most frequently at the nape of the neck (Figure 7.31). Hypertrophic scars, keloid scarring and alopecia develop in the same area (Figure 7.32). The pustules are usually sterile, and the etiology is thought to involve curving and inward growth of corkscrew-shaped hairs. Treatment is difficult, but systemic antibiotics may afford temporary relief, and intralesional steroid injections help to flatten the keloid scars.

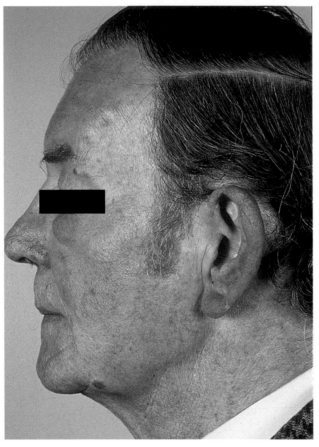

Figure 7.28

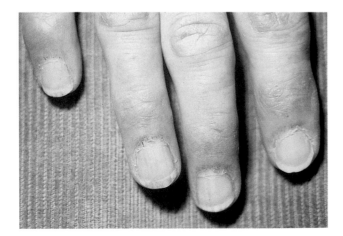

Figure 7.29

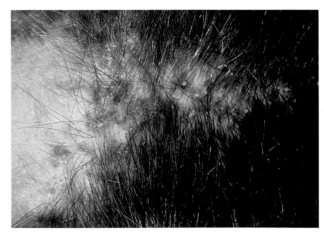

Figure 7.30

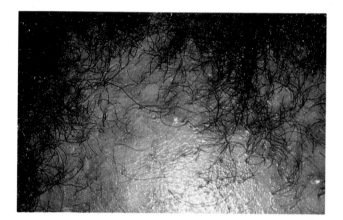

Figure 7.31

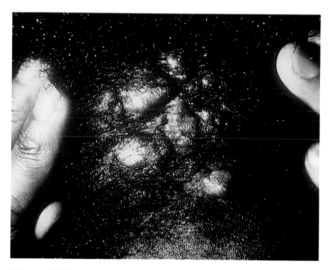

Figure 7.32

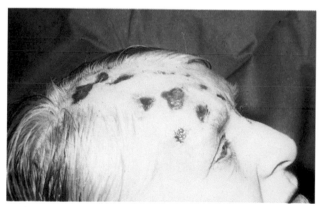

Figure 7.33

POST-ZOSTER EROSIONS

One of the complications following herpes zoster (shingles) is dysesthesia. This may lead to artefactual 'picking' of lesions in the area and non-healing erosions as seen in Figure 7.33 following shingles of the ophthalmic division of the trigeminal nerve.

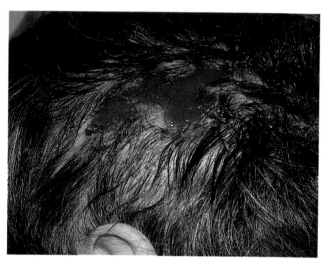

Figure 7.34

GIANT CELL ARTERITIS

Giant cell arteritis (temporal arteritis) is of unknown etiology and affects elderly patients of both sexes. It is important to treat this early with systemic antibiotics because, if left untreated, there is a risk of blindness. It may also cause inflammation and erosions of the skin in the area of the temporal artery (Figure 7.34), with secondary alopecia.

OTHER DERMATOSES

Other dermatoses which cause cicatricial alopecia have been discussed earlier in Chapter 3. These comprise lupus erythematosus, lichen planus, cicatricial pemphigoid, morphea and scleroderma.

REFERENCES

1. Schuster S, Blatchford N. *Seborrhoeic Dermatitis and Dandruff – a Fungal Disease*. London: Royal Society of Medicine Publishing, 1988
2. Ring DS, Kaplan DL. Pityriasis amiantacea: a report of 10 cases. *Arch Dermatol* 1993;129:913–15
3. Wilkinson J. Contact dermatitis. *Dermatol Pract* 1982;Aug:8–15
4. Dawber RPR. Aspects of treatment of scalp psoriasis. *J Dermatol Treat* 1989;1:1
5. Burge S, Wilkinson JD. Darier's disease: a clinical study. *Br J Dermatol* 1991;125:14
6. Pye RJ, Peachey RDC, Burton JL. Erosive pustular dermatosis of the scalp. *Br J Dermatol* 1979;100:559–61

8

Scalp tumors

CYSTS

Epidermoid cysts

Epidermoid (epidermal) cysts, although often misnamed sebaceous cysts, are, indeed, of epidermal origin. They are extremely common in adults and clinically appear as smooth, domed lesions, mobile over underlying tissues (Figure 8.1). They often have a visible central punctum, express cheesy keratin material when traumatized and can become secondarily infected. Histologically, the wall of the cyst is formed by keratinizing squamous epithelium, which fills the cyst cavity with layers of keratin. Treatment is by simple excision under local anesthetic.

Tricholemmal cysts

Tricholemmal cysts (pilar cysts) are similar to epidermoid cysts but are derived from external hair root sheaths and almost always occur on the scalp. They form smooth, firm, mobile nodules (Figure 8.2a) which may distort hair growth (Figure 8.2b) and have a tendency to become secondarily infected. They do not have a central punctum. They are famil-

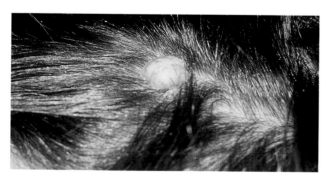

Figure 8.1

ial and more common in women. Histologically, the cyst wall comprises an outer layer of cuboidal cells which merge with an inner layer of eosinophilic cells, which desquamate to form the granular cyst contents.

Congenital inclusion dermoid cysts

Dermoid cysts arise from epithelial cells sequestered in the dermis along lines of embryonic fusion. A classical site is the upper outer corner of the eye. The cysts may be superficial and palpable or lie deep. Deeper cysts may present as a focal area of aplasia cutis (Figure 8.3). Histologically, they comprise squamous epithelium and adnexal structures and the cyst cavity is often filled with hair. Dermoid cysts may be difficult to excise owing to deep tracts adhered to underlying periosteum. They must be carefully distinguished from meningoencephaloceles or nasal gliomas and should be investigated radiologically prior to surgical intervention.

Heterotropic brain tissue cysts

Lesions of heterotropic brain tissue may present as soft nodules on the scalp. They are classically surrounded by a collar of hair (Figure 8.4).

NEVI

Epidermal nevi

Epidermal nevi are benign lesions which are either present at birth or arise in the first decade of life. There are several clinical subtypes including nevus verrucous, which presents as a warty yellow/brown

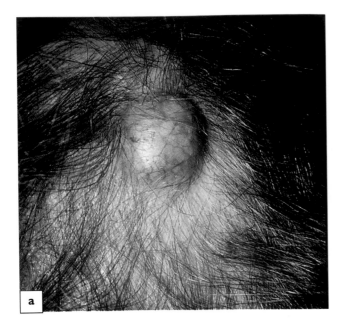

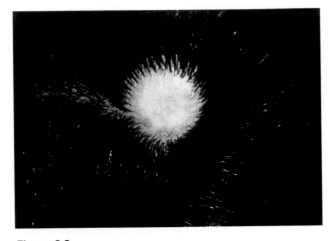

Figure 8.3

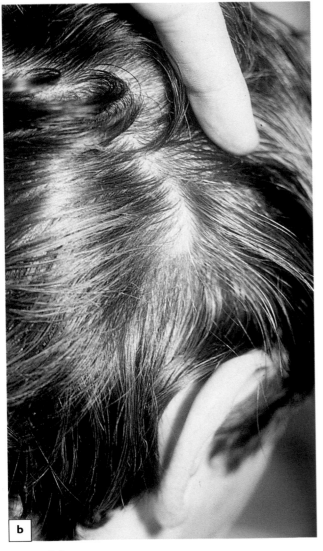

Figure 8.2

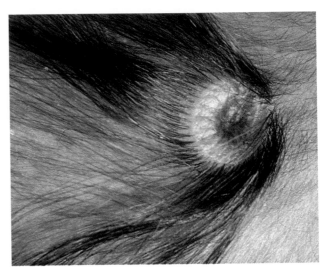

Figure 8.4

plaque (Figure 8.5a), and linear epidermal nevi (Figure 8.5b). They can occur on the scalp and may be misdiagnosed as a seborrheic wart. The epidermal nevus syndrome is the association of a widespread epidermal nevus with skeletal, ocular and/or cerebral defects. Histologically, they vary but generally have hyperkeratosis, papillomatosis and acanthosis.

Sebaceous nevi

Sebaceous nevi (or organoid nevi) are hamartomas comprised mainly of sebaceous glands. Clinically, they appear as single, well-defined, pink or yellow velvety non-hair-bearing plaques, classically on the scalp or face (Figure 8.6a). The lesions become less prominent following birth but thicken again at puberty owing to hormonal effects on the sebaceous glands. Histologically, they vary but usually have an acanthotic, papillomatous epithelium with increased

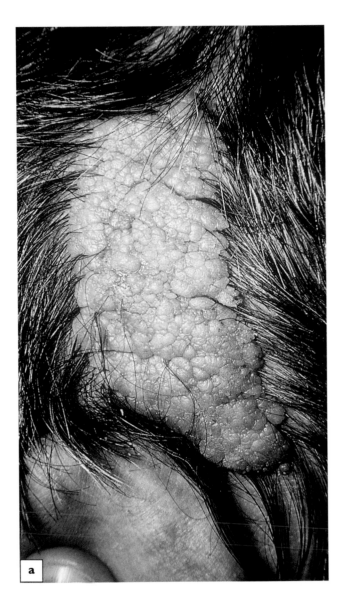

numbers of distorted sebaceous glands in the dermis. Many different tumors may develop within these nevi. The majority are benign, but basal cell carcinomas (Figure 8.6b) and, very rarely, squamous cell carcinomas are reported. Because of this small risk, sebaceous nevi should be prophylactically excised when the patient is at a suitable age.

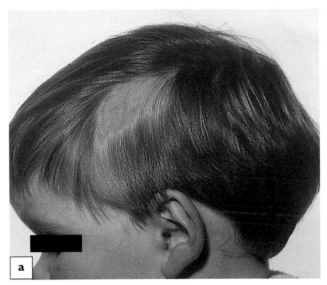

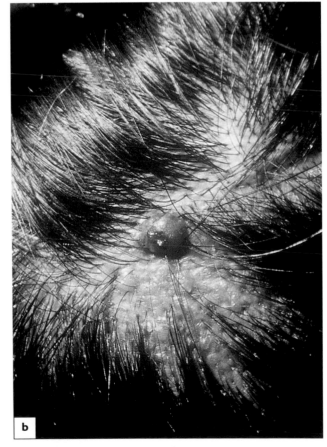

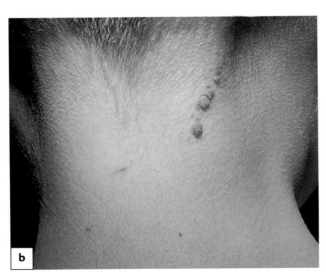

Figure 8.5

Figure 8.6

Syringocystadenoma papilliferum

This is a nevus derived from apocrine sweat glands. It presents as a single or multiple erythematous nodule(s) either at or soon after birth. They can form plaques or linear groups of lesions (Figure 8.7) and often arise within sebaceous nevi. Approximately 10% go on to develop a basal cell carcinoma. Histologically, they are composed of two cell types forming papillae connected by ducts, with an inner lining of columnar cells and an outer layer of cuboidal cells.

Strawberry nevus

Strawberry nevi (capillary hemangiomae) are benign vascular tumors. They almost always appear during the first month of infancy, with a prevalence of approximately 3%. At birth, they are often absent, appearing a few days later as a macular area of hyperemia. Lesions typically enlarge over a number of weeks to form the classic 'strawberry' and eventually spontaneously regress, with an estimated 50% resolved by the age of 5 years. They can occur at any site, but are most commonly seen on the head and neck (Figure 8.8). Superficial lesions have a better chance of complete resolution than deeper lesions. Histologically, they represent a proliferation of small vascular channels lined with plump endothelial cells.

Uncomplicated lesions are usually left to resolve spontaneously. Lesions occurring at important sites such as near the eye, mouth or anus can interfere with function and may need to be treated. Rapidly expanding lesions may be treated with oral steroids. Established nevi or early hyperemic patches may be treated with a vascular laser.

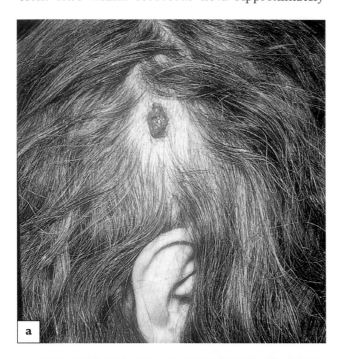

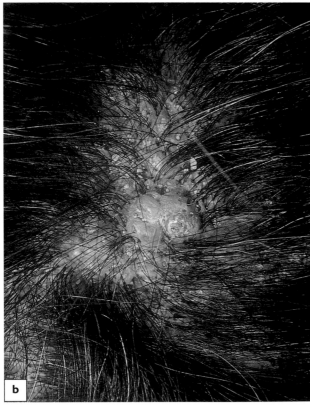

Figure 8.7

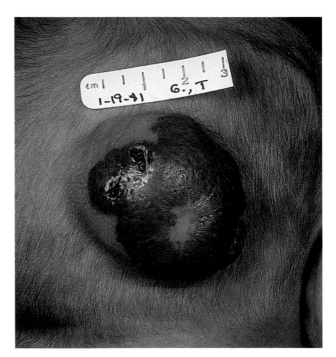

Figure 8.8

Capillary vascular malformations

Capillary vascular malformations of the so-called 'salmon patch' variety are extremely common telangiectatic nevi which are usually present at birth. They appear as dull red, irregular, macular areas, often on the face, where they fade, but most commonly at the nape of the neck, where they are more persistent (Figure 8.9).

Capillary vascular malformations of the so-called 'port wine stain' variety, or nevus flammeus, are permanent telangiectatic nevi which are usually present at birth. They most commonly affect the face and vary in color from pink to red (Figure 8.10).

Vascular ocular abnormalities can occur in association with them if the periorbital area is affected. 'Port wine stains' affecting the trigeminal distribution may be associated with cerebral angiomatosis, forming the Sturge–Weber syndrome. Histologically, they are composed of numerous thin-walled vascular channels.

Melanocytic nevi

Melanocytic nevi are proliferations of melanocytes at the dermal–epidermal junction, which usually occur in small clusters called 'nests'. Lesions mature with age and nests of melanocytes migrate into the dermis. Lesions with nests only at the dermal–epidermal junction are called junctional nevi. Lesions with a mixture of nests at the junction and deeper in the dermis are termed compound nevi and lesions purely with nests in the dermis are intradermal nevi. Benign intradermal and compound melanocytic nevi occur commonly on the face and scalp (see Chapter 4, Figure 4.7), but malignant melanomas are rare. Blue nevi are a variant in which melanocytes have a spindle-shaped histologic appearance and lie deep in the dermis. Clinically, they have a characteristic dusky blue/black appearance (Figure 8.11). Spitz's nevi (juvenile melanomas) are benign compound nevi which present as red/brown or pink-colored nodules.

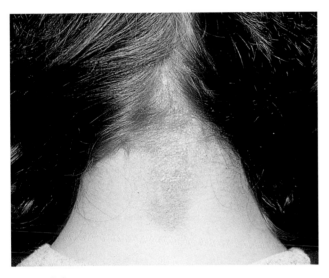

Figure 8.9

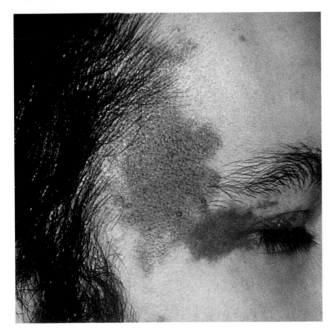

Figure 8.10

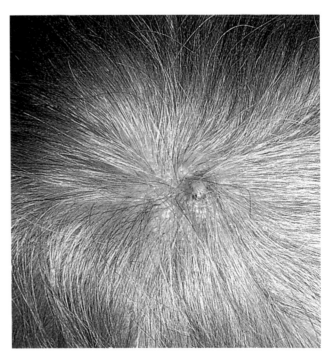

Figure 8.11

Histologically, they have spindle- or polygonal-shaped melanocytes arranged in nests or cords, with abundant eosinophilic cytoplasm. They are often associated with multiple giant cells. Blue nevi and Spitz's nevi occur as commonly on the scalp as elsewhere.

BENIGN TUMORS

Seborrheic keratosis

Seborrheic keratosis (seborrheic warts, basal cell papillomas) are common benign epidermal lesions that can occur at any site, including the scalp. Clinically, they have a 'stuck on' appearance, with characteristic fissuring of the surface (Figure 8.12). They are unusual in childhood but become increasingly common from middle age onwards. Histologically, they are tumors of epidermal basal cells with keratin cysts, and many different patterns are recognized. They may be left alone, but, if they become recurrently traumatized and/or irritated, treatment with curettage and cautery or cryotherapy may be warranted.

Solar keratosis

Solar keratoses (actinic keratoses) are found at sites exposed to sun and occur commonly on bald scalps (Figure 8.13). They appear as rough, scaly superficial patches that may crust recurrently and represent areas of epidermal dysplasia. Multiple lesions are often present. Histologically, the epidermis is parakeratotic and loses its granular layer. The

keratinocytes show varying degrees of dysplasia. Solar keratoses may resolve spontaneously or be treated with numerous methods including cryotherapy, curettage and cautery, or topical 5-fluorouracil cream. However, they may be the precursor to a squamous cell carcinoma; thus solar keratoses which have become more indurated should be biopsied in case of malignant change (Figure 8.14).

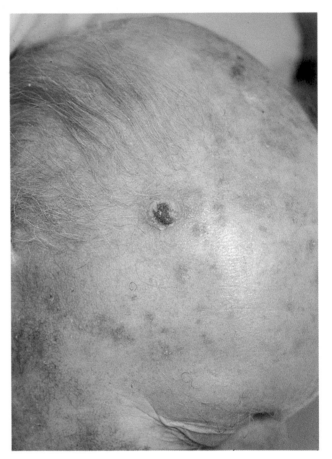

Figure 8.13

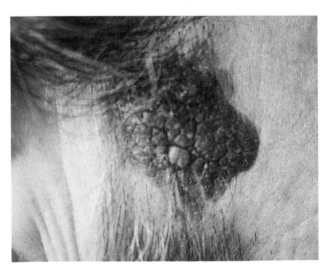

Figure 8.12

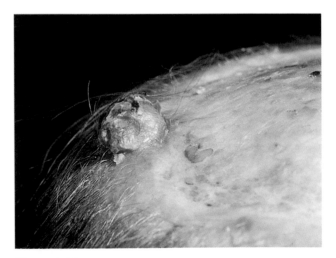

Figure 8.14

Keratoacanthoma

Keratoacanthomas are common tumors which occur mainly on sites exposed to sun, in older people. They are rapidly growing and resolve spontaneously to leave a pit-like scar. They classically form smooth-shouldered tumors with a central keratin plug (Figure 8.15). The main differential diagnosis both clinically and histologically is a squamous cell carcinoma. Histologically, the keratin horn is symmetrically surrounded by acanthotic epithelium, with very few mitoses. The base is flattened with no invasion. Lesions may be curetted or excised.

Pilomatricoma

Pilomatricoma (calcifying epithelioma of Malherbe) are benign tumors derived from hair matrix cells occuring in hair-bearing areas (Figure 8.16). They usually present in childhood as a dermal nodule or a subcutaneous calcified lesion, characterized by its stone-hard consistency. The histology is distinctive, with areas of peripheral basophilic cells which develop abundant eosinophilic cytoplasm towards the center of the lesion. The basophilic material disappears and nuclear outlines remain to form 'ghost cells'. Malignant pilomatricomas are rare.

Trichofolliculoma

These are uncommon hamartomas of the pilosebaceous unit, which form small facial nodules with hair protruding in a tuft (Figure 8.17). Histologically, they form a large, dilated, pilosebaceous canal with several pilosebaceous units attached. Central hair shafts are often present, and are seen well with polarized light.

Trichoepithelioma

This is a hamartoma of the pilosebaceous unit which occurs more deeply in the dermis than the trichofolliculoma. They are often familial and may be associated with cylindromas to form the Brooke–Speigler syndrome. Clinically and histologically, they may resemble a basal cell carcinoma. Lesions are shiny, with telangiectasia and most commonly occur on the face (Figure 8.18). Histologically, they comprise basophilic cells which form pallisaded lobules and surround eosinophilic amorphous material.

Cylindroma

Cylindroma ('turban tumors') are benign tumors of uncertain origin, which most commonly occur on the scalp. They form slow-growing, smooth, red/pink

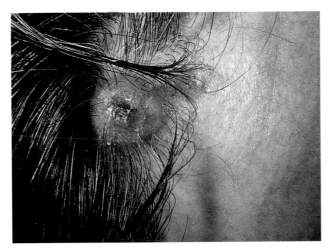

Figure 8.15

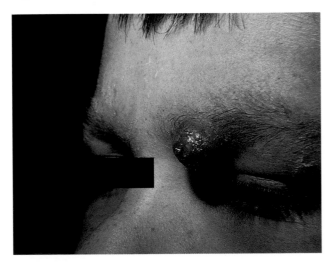

Figure 8.16

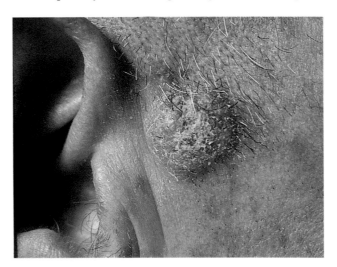

Figure 8.17

nodules which may be pedunculated (Figure 8.19). Lesions may be multiple, and familial cases are reported. When multiple cylindromas occur on the scalp, they are sometimes described as the 'turban' tumor. Histology is distinctive, with lobules of basophilic cells, surrounding duct-like spaces and surrounded by eosinophilic hyaline material. The lobules are arranged in a 'jigsaw-type' pattern.

Pyogenic granuloma

Pyogenic granulomas are extremely common benign proliferations of vascular tissue which arise following trauma to the skin. They are friable, red/purple nodules which tend to bleed. They are most common on the fingers but can occur on the face or scalp (Figure 8.20).

Angiolymphoid hyperplasia with eosinophilia

Angiolymphoid hyperplasia with eosinophilia (Kimura's disease) is a benign, proliferating, vascular condition which affects middle-aged adults and is more common in women. It presents as vascular, dome-shaped nodules often affecting the scalp or ear (Figure 8.21). It is much more common in Japan. Kimura's disease is now thought to represent a similar but separate entity where lesions occur more

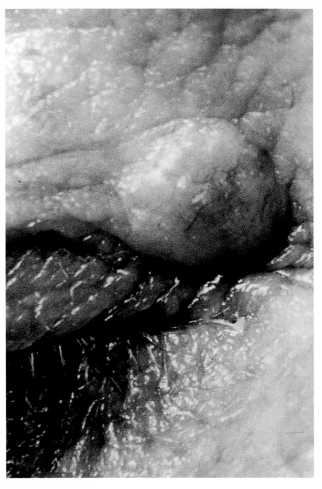

Figure 8.18

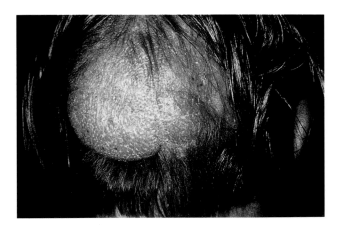

Figure 8.19

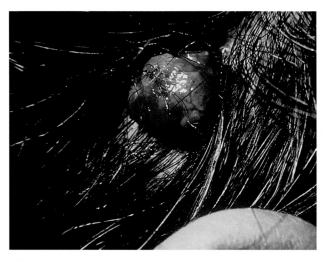

Figure 8.20

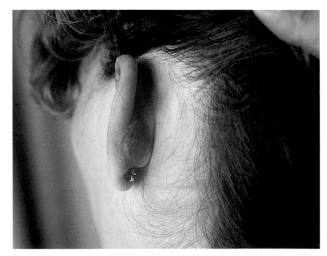

Figure 8.21

deeply and may have an associated peripheral eosinophilia. Histologically, they appear as disorganized groups of proliferating capillaries with a lymphocytic and eosinophilic infiltrate. Excision is the treatment of choice.

Atypical fibroxanthoma

Atypical fibroxanthomata classically arise in the elderly, on sites exposed to the sun. They present as enlarging, red, fleshy tumors (Figure 8.22) and have a worrying histologic appearance, with atypical giant cells and many mitoses. Paradoxically, their clinical behavior is benign and limited local excision should provide adequate treatment.

MALIGNANT TUMORS

Basal cell carcinomas

These common tumors usually arise on the scalp of patients with thinned hair, owing to excessive exposure to the sun (Figure 8.23). In one series, 5% of basal cell carcinomas occurred on the scalp. Patients who previously received X-ray depilation for scalp ringworm are at particular risk (Figure 8.24). Large neglected lesions may invade periosteum or bone. Their appearance is the same as at other sites, often forming a crusted lesion with a rolled, shiny, pearly edge (Figure 8.25). Nodules often have overlying

telangiectasia. Morpheic basal cell carcinomas also occur on the scalp.

Squamous cell carcinomas

Squamous cell carcinomas on the scalp may be fast growing and present as large, crusted indurated lesions (Figure 8.26). They often arise from existing

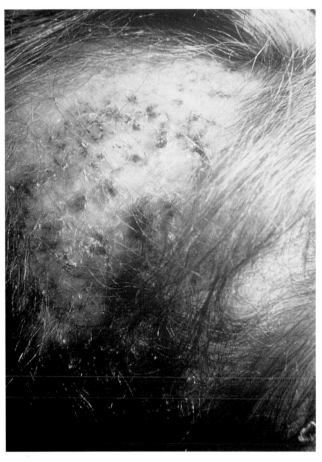

Figure 8.23

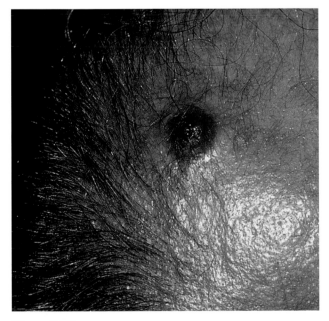

Figure 8.22

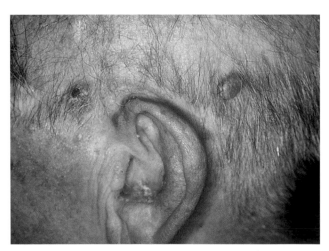

Figure 8.24

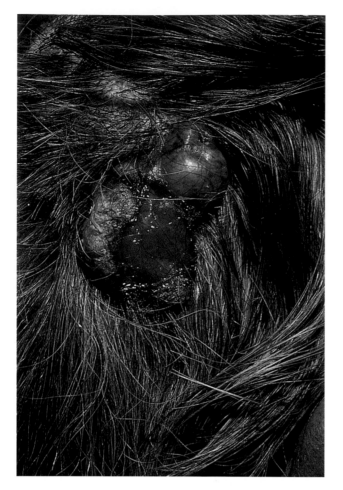

Figure 8.25

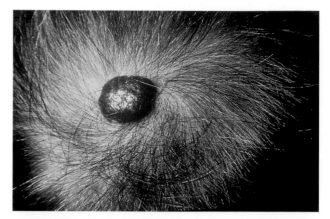

Figure 8.27

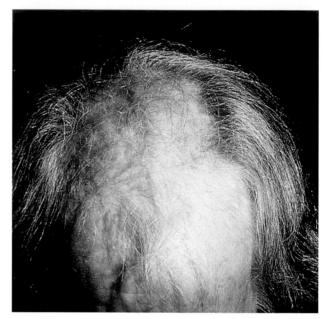

Figure 8.28

Cutaneous metastases to the scalp

The scalp is a common site for cutaneous metastases, particularly from renal or breast carcinoma. They present as firm, single (Figure 8.27) or multiple, rapidly expanding nodules. Cutaneous metastasis may be the presenting sign of an underlying carcinoma. Metastases to the scalp can induce a fibrotic reaction pattern which presents as a scarring alopecia, termed 'alopecia neoplastica' (Figure 8.28). Histology of the metastases may resemble the tumor of origin or may be too anaplastic to identify.

Angiosarcoma

Angiosarcoma generally presents in the elderly population and is seen more commonly in men. Lesions often present as groups of red/blue nodules

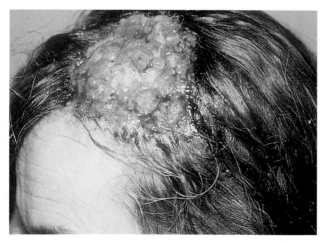

Figure 8.26

solar keratoses in patients with thinning hair; thus solar keratoses which have become more indurated should be biopsied in case of malignant change. Previous use of X-ray depilation of the scalp to treat ringworm infection is a risk factor for developing squamous cell carcinoma.

on the face or scalp, although less commonly they present as a banal-looking bruise on the scalp (Figure 8.29). Histologically, they form anastomosing vascular channels lined with atypical endothelial cells. They behave aggressively, with an average survival of

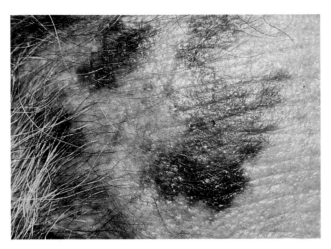

Figure 8.29

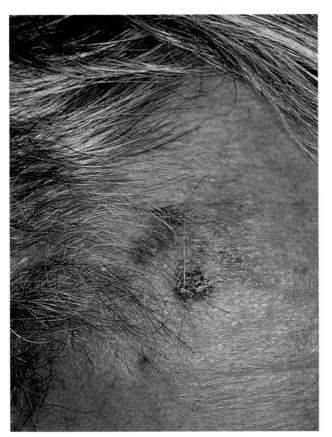

Figure 8.30

2 years following diagnosis. They are resistant to most treatments, but palliative radiotherapy may help.

Lentigo maligna

Lentigo maligna (or Hutchinson's freckle) is a slow-growing, horizontal proliferation of atypical melanocytes. It most commonly present on the face or scalp of the elderly, as a macule with irregular pigmentation and/or shape (Figure 8.30). Untreated lesions may in time become invasive, often with formation of nodules within the lesion, and be termed a lentigo maligna melanoma.

REFERENCES

1. Pinkus H. Sebaceous cysts are tricholemmal cysts. *Arch Dermatol* 1969;99:544
2. Sinclair R, Darley C, Dawber RPR. Congenital inclusion dermoid cyst of the scalp. *Aust J Dermatol* 1992;33:135
3. Wilson Jones E, Bleehan SS. Inflammatory angiomatous nodules with abnormal blood vessels occurring about the ears and scalp. *Br J Dermatol* 1969;81:804
4. Bowers RE, Graham EA, Tomlinson KM. The natural history of the strawberry naevus. *Arch Dermatol* 1960;82:167
5. Holden CA, Spittle MF, Jones FW. Angiosarcoma of the face and scalp: prognosis and treatment. *Cancer* 1987;59:1046
6. Mehegran AH. Metastatic carcinoma to the skin. *Dermatologica* 1961;123:311
7. Pinkus H, Sutton RL. Trichofolliculoma. *Arch Dermatol* 1965;91:46
8. Cerroni L, Salmhofer W, Hodl S. Clinical and histological spectrum of pilomatrixomas in adults. *Int J Dermatol* 1994;33:705
9. Rook A, Whimster I. Keratoacanthoma – a 30 year retrospect. *Br J Dermatol* 1979;100:41
10. Fergin PE, Chu AC, Macdonald DM. Basal cell carcinoma complicating naevus sebaceous. *Clin Exp Dermatol* 1981;6:111
11. Jancar J. Naevus syringocystadenomatosus papilliferus. *Br J Dermatol* 1970;82:402
12. Delfino M, D'anna F, Ianniello S, Donofrio V. Multiple hereditary trichoepitheliomas and cylindromas (Brooke–Speigler syndrome). *Dermatologica* 1991;183:150–3

9

Chemical and physical hair damage

SHAMPOOS AND CONDITIONERS

Shampoos basically contain principal surfactants to foam and act as a detergent, secondary surfactants to condition the hair, and additives for specific reasons, e.g. vitamins or herbal extracts. Conditioners contain fatty acids and alcohols which aim to make hair shiny and lubricate it to make combing easier. Shampoos all contain detergents and are therefore potential contact irritants. This is usually only a problem for patients with atopic eczema or people who are in prolonged contact with shampoos, e.g. hairdressers, in whom they can cause irritant hand dermatitis. Allergic contact dermatitis can occur to fragrance, formaldehyde and biocides within shampoos and conditioners. Excessive use of shampoos and lack of conditioning can lead to increased weathering of the hair.

Sudden, irreversible matting and tangling of the hair has been reported secondary to the use of shampoos (Figure 9.1a), and been given the name 'bird's nest hair'. Electron microscopy of matted hair reveals welding of the hairs, which has occurred via a process of 'felting' (Figure 9.1b).

HAIR COLORING – DYES AND BLEACHES

Hair dyes are divided into three types, vegetable, metallic and synthetic organic materials. The traditional vegetable dye is henna which gives a red/auburn color. Mixing henna with indigo leaves forms darker blue/black dyes. The recent fashion for using henna for temporary skin tattooing has highlighted the potential risk of allergic contact dermatitis with this chemical, although the paraphenylenediamine (PPD) mixed with the henna is the usual

culprit. Camomile contains a yellow dye and is traditionally used to lighten/brighten blonde hair. It can also cause a contact allergy. Metallic dyes gradually change hair color, leaving a dulled appearance and causing weathering if used in excess. Synthetic organic dyes can be temporary, semi-permanent or permanent. Permanent dyes require the additional use of hydrogen peroxide, as an oxidizing agent, in order to produce their final color, a process which can cause much weathering of the hair. PPD is a common permanent dye used for dark/black shades.

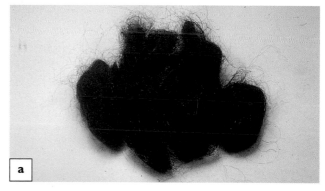

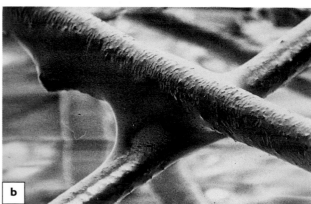

Figure 9.1

It is also a common contact allergen, affecting up to 10% of people who use it (Figure 9.2, see also Figure 7.14).

Hydrogen peroxide is used to oxidize melanin and cause bleaching of the hair for lighter shades. Its use can leave dark hair with a red tinge. The hair becomes more porous, and overuse can cause marked weathering with dryness, brittleness and easy tangling (Figure 9.3). Weathering caused by acute bleach damage can be dramatically seen via electron microscopy of the hair shaft (Figure 9.4).

HAIR WAVING AND STRAIGHTENING

Steam is able to disrupt keratin disulfide bonds and has traditionally been used to create temporary waves in hair. Permanent waving involves softening of the hair, physical reshaping and hardening again to retain the new shape. 'Perming' can cause much weathering of the hair shaft, as demonstrated on electron microscopy (Figure 9.5). Softening lotions often contain thioglycolate with ammonia or glyceryl monothioglycolate to reduce disulfide bonds. Curlers are used to physically shape the hair and hardeners, often hydrogen peroxide, are then applied to oxidize the disulfide bonds again. Allergic contact dermatitis to glyceryl monothioglycolate is increasingly common in hairdressers.

'Hot combing' is a method of applying heat to straighten hair. Misuse can cause a scarring alopecia (Figure 9.6). High temperatures from faulty hair dryers can lead to the development of 'bubble hair'

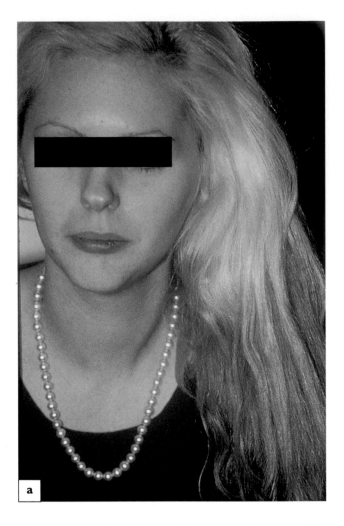

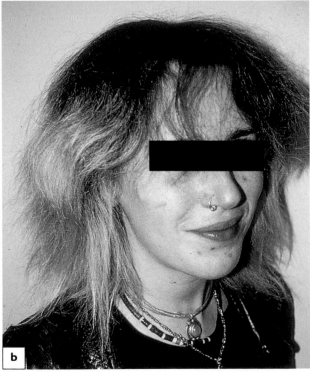

Figure 9.2

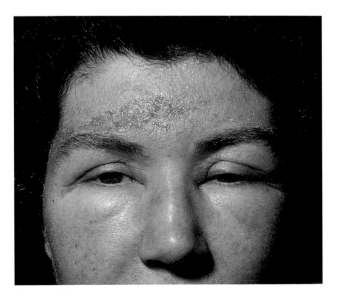

Figure 9.3

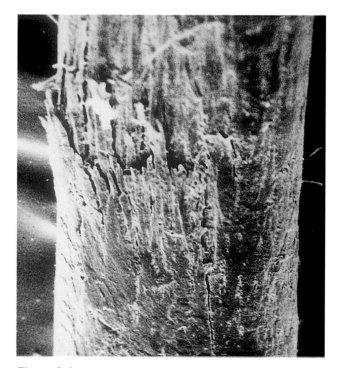

Figure 9.4

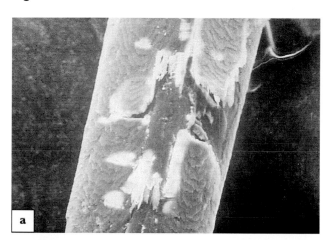

a

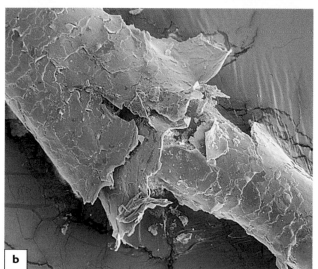

b

Figure 9.5

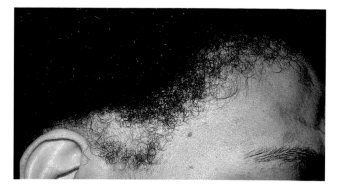

Figure 9.6

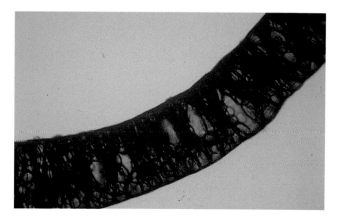

Figure 9.7

(Figure 9.7), probably owing to the rapid vaporization of water within the hair shaft.

PHYSICAL TREATMENTS

Repeated back-combing and brushing of hair can in itself cause marked weathering (Figure 9.8). Repeated styling of hair where roots are placed under tension can lead to the development of traction alopecia, seen with the hair style in place (Figure 9.9), and persisting when the hair style is no longer worn, years later (Figure 9.10).

TRICHOTILLOMANIA

Trichotillomania is the compulsive plucking and pulling of a patient's own hair. It occurs twice as commonly in adult women than adult men, and is also seen in children, where the frontal scalp is most commonly affected (Figure 9.11). Patients classically present with an area of plucked, uniformly short, stubbly hairs, of approximately 3 mm length, with normal hair at the margins. The most common

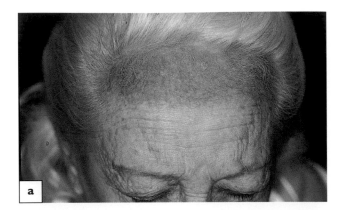

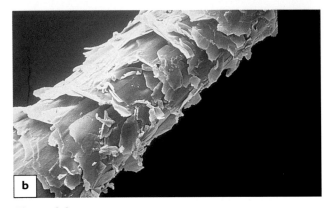

Figure 9.8

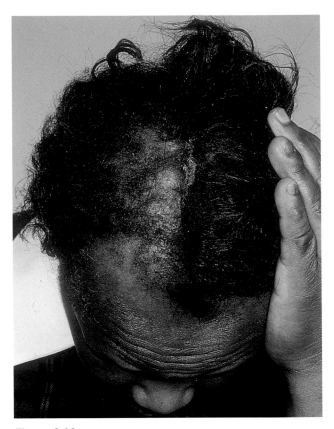

Figure 9.10

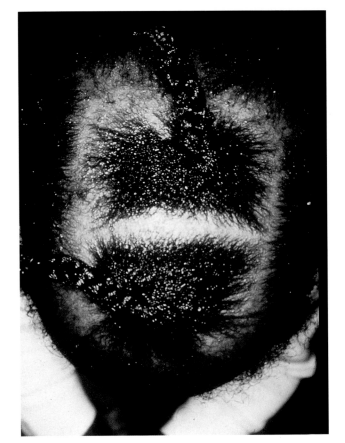

Figure 9.9

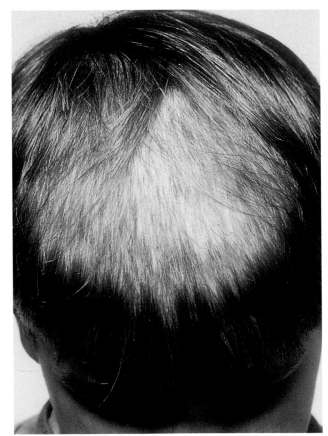

Figure 9.11

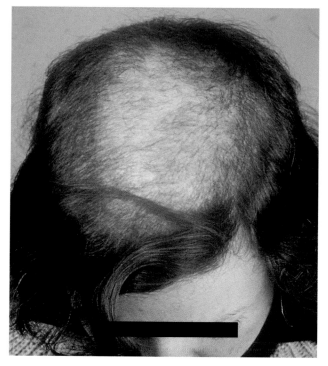

Figure 9.12

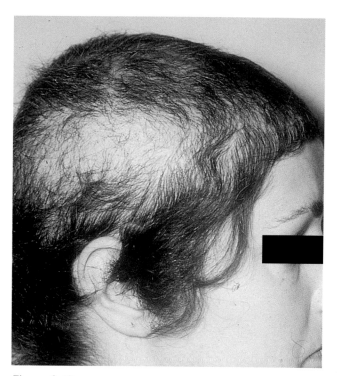

Figure 9.13

pattern is of central scalp loss of hair – the 'tonsure' pattern (Figure 9.12), and may be unilateral (Figure 9.13). The prognosis for recovery in adults is poor.

REFERENCES

1. Wilkinson JB, Moore RJ, eds. *Harry's Cosmetology*, 7th edn. London: Longman Scientific and Technical, 1982

2. Zviak C, Camp M, eds. *The Science of Hair Care*. New York: Marcel Dekker, 1986

3. Dawber RPR, Calnan CD. Bird's nest hair – matting of scalp hair due to shampooing. *Clin Exp Dermatol* 1976;1:155

4. Dawber RPR, ed. *Shampoos – Scientific Basis and Clinical Aspects*. Int Congress and Symposium Series 1995;216

5. Baran R, Maibach HI, eds. *Cosmetic Dermatology*. London: Martin Dunitz Ltd., 1998

Index